MY POWER DECADE

A STORY OF MINDSET, WEIGHT LOSS, MUSCLE GAIN, & RECLAIMING HEALTH AFTER AGE SIXTY

JULIA LINN

ISBN: 978-1-64184-877-0 (Hardcover)
ISBN: 978-1-64184-883-1 (Paperback)
ISBN: 978-1-64184-884-8 (Ebook)

I dedicate this book to Paul

ACKNOWLEDGEMENTS

My fullest gratitude goes to God, Holy Spirit, the Ancient of Days, the Creator, the ONE, Divine Love, Allah, Source, the All in All. There are so many names and yet it feels unnameable, nameless.

I am grateful to my parents who agreed to bring me here and do the best they could in my life, all four of my grandparents who were courageous beings in their own right. I am deeply grateful to my organ donor Gina who died in a car accident when she was 25 in Colorado. Her donated tissue and organs blessed up to 70 people.

Her kidney and pancreas were the gift of life to me.

I'm grateful to my husband's daughter, Lauren, who allowed me to be in her life as a parent and a friend.

I'm grateful for all the friends I have made around the world over the decades at different stages of my life, the students I have taught, the people in the fitness world who have encouraged me and coached me, like my friend David Coleman and his wife Jennifer. I'm grateful for Tom Bird, my writing coach and the amazing Queenagers who follow me on Instagram and share their stories with me.

I'm the most grateful to my husband Paul for his undying love and support under any conditions since 1988. He knows how to make my life a safe, loving, peaceful place, especially when I have been too weak to be strong. I love you so much, Paulji.

PREFACE

Hello, my lovely Queenager!

You might think this book is about me, but it's really about you: A woman coming into her power in her 60's who wants to realize what her entire life has prepared her for. She is inside of you waiting to be released. I call this time The Power Decade but truly, it's The Love Decade. The decade you decide to finally love and care for yourself, after taking care of others your whole life. Now you know you can't give from an empty cup.

The narrative of the "older" woman ignores that we have *gotten things done.* We multi-task, care-give, work hard, love hard, dream big, and find a way to be a badass from here to Sunday. We are powerful.

We've had hardships, courtships, fellowships, mentorships, and kinships! You are the wisdom keepers and must share your genius with the world!

I'm telling you my whole story so you can see yours in mine. With all the drama, messiness, low self-esteem, self-loathing, poor choices, vulnerabilities, triumphs, love, loss, hope, and courage.

Our bodies are a chariot for the Soul. That chariot can be a bit shopworn when we hit 60. Mine was. At 62 I felt stuck, sluggish, and wore the body of a very out-of-shape 62-year-old.

I decided it was not going to be another chapter in the diet wars, with my body the repository of frustrations, deprivation, and the weaponizing of food.

I found my WHY to get optimally healthy. A big, big WHY. And then ... BANG BANG!

I became a SHAPESHIFTER, and in a nanosecond made a mind shift to who I KNEW I really was. I became the real ME, with all the energy I needed to continue to live my life feeling amazing! She was just waiting for this moment to arrive.

It was not about my body. It was about my spirit and my mindset and SHAPESHIFTING there, and how it *manifested* in my body. What became my Power Decade started with Love – self-love.

This is not a "How to" diet or fitness book. This book is a mirror reflecting back to you feelings women have had who are close to, in, or beyond age 60. What's possible? Everything!

No matter where you live in the world, you are my sister and I share my story with you in that light. Nothing held back.

The "How Come" of this story will soon be followed by a "How To." I know and believe with all my heart that if I can transform – you can too! And the next book will give you all the steps I followed to get in the best shape of my life, in body, mind and spirit.

With love and cheers,

Julia Linn
February 2023

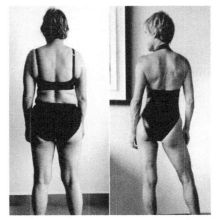

Julia Linn, 2019 and 2023

CHAPTERS

ONE

HELLO, DEATH, NOT SO NICE
TO MEET YOU

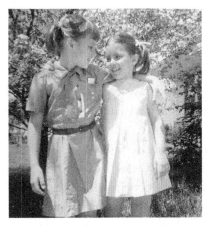

Nancy Adore, 1960 – 1966

L ying by the hotel pool in the sun, watching light sparkle on the water, I was jarred by the shadow created by a man standing over me.

"I really loved your presentation," he said.

I shaded my eyes against the sun and immediately registered his attractiveness. My thoughts flew to my lumpy thighs. *Oh god, if I cover myself with a towel right now, will my shame be obvious?*

He talked on. I'm wondering why an attractive man would want to talk to me, a woman in her early 40's with lumpy thighs, lying by the pool. Forget that my presentation had moved him (and many others I heard from while wearing regular attire) and there was zero energy of a come-on.

The truth was: I hated my body. Especially my thighs. And oh, I had good reason. All this corporeal disruption and self-loathing of my body started early. So did the disruption of my emotional, mental, and spiritual selves . . . .

It was 1969, and I was crying in my 1960's decorated bedroom with my stuffed animals and Beatles posters on the walls. There was a little sign I cut out of a magazine and taped to my silver chrome lamp. It said: "All she wants is pierced ears and blonde hair." That was me at 11.

But a bomb had exploded in my family – twice in three years. First my younger sister died of cancer after suffering for a full year. I was 9. Two years later, I was diagnosed with Type 1 diabetes. Pierced ears and blonde hair seemed so incredibly stupid and trivial.

Now what I wanted was for Jesus to make an appearance – because my sister had died and I didn't understand why and she was only 6 years old. She suffered so much. We all watched her suffer, it was awful; and within a year this beautiful dark-haired child was gone. At age 9, I wanted to know where did she go? Why did she go? Why did God take her and she only got 6 years of life?

I was told God works in mysterious ways, but I wanted to know those ways – why why why? – and I was told she was in heaven because she was baptized. I thought, *What about all those little brown children who live in the forest who have never heard of Jesus? Do they go to hell?* I could not believe that God would be so unfair.

So, two years later, at age 11, in my polka dot, striped black and white bedroom with bright orange pops of color and my chrome lamp and my Beatles posters, I challenged this Jesus to make an appearance. Not only was my sister taken away, but just two years after Nancy died, I got diabetes. It devastated me.

I thought where is the Jesus that's supposed to love and protect me? Where is the presence I always felt was with me; but not now? I challenged Jesus to prove his realness and his presence as I sat in the dark that night on my bed, waiting for something to happen; a stuffed animal to fall off the shelf, anything to prove he was real. But nothing happened. Nothing. Nothing at all.

I looked out my second-floor bedroom window to the dark backyard. The yard ended on the edge of a ravine behind our house. I looked at all the trees and felt the desolation, anger, and abrupt absence of a belief I'd had since I was a young child. That Jesus loves me this I know because the Bible told me so. But I didn't believe it now nor would I ever again. The dark backyard reflected my feelings of betrayal. The intensity of my anger with this lack of spiritual proof was the reason I told my parents at age 12: I am never going back to church!

We lived on a cul-de-sac in West Lafayette, Indiana, in a manicured, middle-class modern mid-century split-level, with a two-car garage, slate floor foyer, sunken living room and early American colonial interior decoration. My parents had designed and built the home for a large family, as a part of the American Dream. Our household included my parents, four daughters, and our dachshund, Ginger. I was five when we moved in. No one could have predicted four years later family life would shatter. We were oblivious to the coming tsunami of loss and grief with Nancy's illness, an aggressive cancer that was incurable.

After she was stricken, it was a year of blurred memories, since the severity of the situation was kept from us three girls.

We knew Nancy was sick, yet somehow my parents put up a strong front, hiding the tears and sorrow.

After the no-show by Jesus, I would never return to church. It was a place I saw my mother act one way – pious and smiling sweetly — and then get home and act another way, angry and raging. I thought everyone must do that – act one way in church and another way at home. If that was so, I didn't want to return to where the hypocrites were. My mother was always somewhat angry – a woman of the '50s whose own dreams were never realized. Society said you had to marry by 20 – which she did, leaving college to marry my dad. But after Nancy died, the depth of her anger became a rage, despite her ability to go about the motherly duties as expected of her: cooking, cleaning, birthday parties, driving us to sports practice. She did it in a fog of grief, emotionally cut off, without any sense of love. It caused me endless sorrow to think that maybe I was the reason she was always angry. She didn't register the emotional needs and vulnerability of her remaining children. It completely escaped her. She put her head down and just forged ahead with duty.

As a result, I felt unloved and unseen at home. I sought out friends at school and made myself very popular. I don't know how, but I found acceptance and love there that I didn't feel at home. I felt seen.

Before we lost Nancy, we looked like the perfect American family. Four girls, close in age; healthy, young parents; nice house. We would swim all summer at the country club and come home tanned and fit from swim team. The lifeguards loved us. We wore matching bathing suits. Four girls. Three blondes and a dark-haired beauty, third in line, who really stood out. Nancy. Sparkling dark eyes, full of grace and sweetness.

But when we lost Nancy, the world exploded into dark times and years of grief. I cocooned into a space devoid of feeling safe, or cared for. It wasn't possible for my mother to function normally after the death of her 6-year-old daughter. How could she?

My dad was loving and supportive, but he worked a lot. He set up his business so he could indulge his love of golf in the afternoons. We saw him every night for dinner. He'd come home, make a vodka gimlet, and talk to my mom and us about our day. After dinner, he would watch TV in the family room after we all went to bed. Sometimes, though, I would sit on the backrest of the couch with one leg over each of his shoulders, dip a comb in water and comb his hair. It was a way to be with him.

My mom married him at 21 in the 1950s with a lot of ensuing frustration in her life. She put aside her personal goals. Her college education was cut short by choice so she could marry my dad. As years wore on, this manifested as a daily undercurrent of rage, which at times exploded in unpredictable ways.

After my sister died, my mother disappeared into a haze of grief and sorrow that was so deep and wide, she was not available emotionally to her three remaining daughters. My needs were typical of a child that age but on top of that, the unresolved grief and loss was never discussed. My needs were not recognized by my mother at this acute time. My dad was a typical '60s Dad – working a lot, cocktails and dinner at home after work, watching TV until he fell asleep. He was the warm provider of hugs and love, but I went through a period of being angry with him for not protecting me from my mother's rages and rejection.

In fifth grade, two years after my sister died, I was shunned by my close circle of girlfriends. It was December 1968, and the alpha girl in our circle was hell bent on winning a popularity contest organized by the school. You got to ride in the

Christmas parade. I was her biggest competition. I have no idea how she managed to turn all our friends against me. Two months later, I was diagnosed with juvenile onset or Type 1 diabetes. The serious life event[1] of my sister dying and then the diabetes diagnosis was too much for me at 11 – so by 12 I had challenged Jesus.

Two years after Nancy died, my parents announced Mom was pregnant. It suddenly made life more hopeful and brighter. A baby! When my parents brought him home from the hospital, I was struck by his fetal body, curled in on itself with pink skin and a soft mewling cry. He was a treasure! When Bobby arrived, my mother seemed to glow with happiness. I felt like he was mine. I loved to care and play with him — I had just turned 11. He brought such joy into the house. Everyone remarked how much he looked like Nancy. In fact, I felt like Bob was the replacement child for Nancy. As Bobby got older, it was eerie how much they resembled each other. Life seemed to just speed on without any looking back at what had happened before. There was a huge hole inside me from losing Nancy. She was born after me by three years, and her sweet adoration of her big sister – me – caused me endless guilt and pain for all the times I didn't appreciate her unconditional love. There was no one to talk to about any of this. So I just held on with my pre-teen determination. Did what my mom did – head down, forge ahead.

When Bobby was about 10 months old, I remember my mother putting her head down as she leaned on the kitchen counter gathering her thoughts to say something to me. "You are going to the doctor."

---

[1]   Research has shown that serious life events or SLE often precipitate T1diabetes diagnoses in children: https://time.com/3816395/traumatic-life-events-diabetes/

My vision was blurred and my weight had dropped to 60 pounds from 80. I was 11. I was moody all the time and incredibly thirsty. My skin itched. I had no energy or appetite. My parents kept asking me where is the "old Julia?" and I hated that. Later, I realized I was so sick with undiagnosed diabetes but it became a behavioral issue. The blame and guilt I felt for not being the "old Julia" was a burden I couldn't figure out how to lift.

It was early 1969, I was not yet 12. Exhausted, with no energy, I could not drink enough to satisfy this ungodly thirst. I would go down to the basement and raid the refrigerator for orange soda. I was pouring sugar into my body to slake my thirst and accelerating the effects of a non-working pancreas that could not handle the sugar. My body started feeding on itself. I was wasting away. I never wanted to eat. My parents complained to me at the dinner table – "Where's the old Julia?" I felt miserable and had no idea what was happening to me.

The doctor's appointment was scheduled and blood was drawn; I don't remember much else other than my mother insisting I had to go. As a family, we always had dinner together at night.

A few nights later, at the dinner table, the phone rang. My dad got up and answered it in the living room. I could barely hear him saying, "Yes, I understand. I see. Yes." A few more words but no indication of who it was.

My sixth sense kicked in and he came back to the table. I looked at him and said, "I have diabetes, don't I?"

His shocked look told me yes before he said, "Yes, honey you do."

"Am I going to die?"

"No, honey!" he said.

I began to cry. I had no idea what diabetes was.

I'd heard of it one time at a birthday party. One of the girls could not have cake because she had "diabetes." That's all I knew. I'd never heard the word before that. It was rare to get attention in my family, but all the focus was on me at that dinner table. My sisters were silent. Little Bobby was in his high chair.

It was at that moment, 10 months after my brother had been born, that my parents chose to deflect from my bad news with some good news of their own. They must have looked across the table at each other and with an imperceptible nod between them, decided to tell us.

After that, nothing was said about the diabetes diagnosis besides this: Dr. Miller wanted me at the hospital the next morning. I had no idea what to expect, nothing was explained to me. Instead, the mood had changed at the dinner table and my parents looked gleeful.

"Your mom is going to have another baby!" Dad said. Mom was smiling and said, "Due in September!"

My heart sank and I slumped in my chair in defeat and horror. They were lying to me about dying from diabetes! Just like they said we would not lose Nancy after her cancer diagnosis. My mother gave birth to my little brother Bob two years after Nancy died. My brother replaced Nancy and now this new baby would replace me. I had not had a moment to process the possibility of my own death when the conversation moved on to who would replace me. Age 11: Unseen. Unheard. Not important. Replaceable.

I was inconsolable but could not express my utter desolation at this revelation. No more was said about the diabetes diagnosis, what it meant, what it was. It was all talk about the new baby coming in September. It was as if I wasn't allowed to be sad, or terrified – Here! Look over here! Ignore that! Not only did my feelings not matter, but my life didn't either.

I knew I was going to die. I began to cry again, but deep down I knew the outcome.

I wasn't going to die.

I went into the hospital for a few weeks while they got my blood sugar under control. They taught me about taking shots of insulin, weighing and calculating my food. The starched white sheets were scratchy and smelled like bleach. A nurse said to my mother, "Your daughter's hair looks like spun gold." I beamed. I never got compliments or attention like that at home. That I remember this 50 years later gives me an indelible, etched, emotionally charged memory.

The medical team arranged for a dietician to educate me on how insulin worked with what I ate. I needed to weigh my food, count calories and pay attention to carbs, fats, and proteins. Stay away from all sugar. Eat at regular times. Avoid insulin reactions or severe hypoglycemia. Don't take your shot without eating, you could go into a coma.

The dietician arrived in my room at the hospital in white, rubber-soled nurses' shoes. There was a swishing sound from her thighs rubbing together as she walked in her white nurse's trousers. She was wearing a white uniform top.

The buttons over her ample bust gaped, struggling to keep closed. She was obese and bursting at the seams. She pulled out sheets of paper with instructions and pictures on them. Pictures of food groups, fruits, vegetables, meats, plus calorie counts, and forbidden foods.

She was telling me I had to weigh all my food and eat at certain times. I could not exceed the caloric intake and carbohydrates had to be closely monitored because they affected the body and the insulin efficiency. Looking at her size, it was hard to believe her — another hypocrite like the church people. Why should I do what she was telling me to do? Did she know what she was talking about?

9

My dad hated shots but he let me practice on him when he came to the hospital. The nurses brought oranges to practice on – but my dad said, "You can practice on me, honey."

I took out a clean syringe, plunged it into the vial of sterile saline, pulled out some fluid, backtracked to get rid of the air in the syringe and he offered up a hairy Dad arm. I swabbed his arm with an alcohol pad, pinched his tricep and carefully injected the sterile saline into his arm. He didn't flinch. My dad was always willing to do that. For me. When I got home it was as if I had been off at camp for the summer for two weeks. No special treatment, no talk about nutrition, no sense of doing anything different from before.

My father was always more in touch with me emotionally, and did what he could to ease the transition to me now being diabetic. He put a small refrigerator in my room that kept my insulin cold. He wanted to buy me a watch with an alarm on it so I'd always wake up at the same time for my shot in the morning. As cool as that sounded, I didn't really want one.

My mom would come into my room in the morning to wake me. She'd take the small insulin vial out of the refrigerator. Then roll it between her hands to stir it up. The glass vial would click against her wedding band. She'd hand me a syringe and leave to make breakfast.

Once my parents saw I had it figured out, and could take shots without a problem, they left me to my own devices and didn't give me much attention regarding my diabetes. There were unspoken expectations in my family that you didn't complain, you did what you had to do, and do not disappoint. The lack of safety around feelings, and expressing genuine emotions, caused me to bottle them up, to be dealt with in therapy as an adult and all the strategies we learn as children that need undoing as adults.

My parents had two babies now to take care of. I felt completely forgotten. At this point, I was on my own and the only person to take care of me was myself. There was no special treatment for me as a diabetic. I took on survival traits both emotionally and physically. I decided I didn't need anyone or anything. That I could do it all on my own. To depend on another was not safe, either for loss of control or the possibility of rejection. My thoughts cemented in ways to guarantee my survival. I was driven at 12 years old to take care of myself. Which as I got into my teens, since I didn't love myself, didn't mean a whole lot.

After I was diagnosed and stabilized, my mother cooked the same as always – homemade desserts after dinner every night – and I was always encouraged to "have some."

"Isn't there sugar in it?"

"Not that much," she would say. I didn't know if it was denial or she just didn't care.

My sweet grandmother, her mother, would visit and make sure to always bake at least one pie with artificial sweetener just for me. She went out of her way to include me in her love and care. Why couldn't my own mother?

My parents were clueless about my 13-year-old life, and not in touch with my pain – they didn't see it. They were too wrapped up in the babies and also had tremendous unresolved grief (and my mom had anger) around my sister's death. Twenty-five years after Nancy died – and we had not been allowed to go to the funeral service – the funeral home that cremated her was moving and doing inventory. Twenty-five years after she died the funeral director called my parents to inquire about what to do with Nancy's cremains – they sat on a shelf for all those years. She would have been 31 by then. Finally, we buried her ashes in a plot that already had engraved stone markers for both my parents. That alone says how deeply the pain was buried and for how long.

At the time, I was so afraid they would go ahead and bury Nancy's ashes without me, since I lived out of state. As usual, I felt disregarded. But we went and were at the graveside.

I was 34 and I laid a rose in Nancy's grave where the tiny urn of ashes was placed. I wept for my sister we lost so long before. I never got to say good-bye to Nancy until that moment, 25 years later.

It had been too painful to think about for my parents or her ashes would not have remained in storage for 25 years. The strategy was to just keep moving forward, find new reasons to live (two more babies) and not stop and reflect. There was nothing in society to help grieving parents – no support groups, no bereavement counseling, no openness about such a tragic loss. People outside and inside the family felt it was best not to talk about it or bring it up.

At age nine, my need to understand death and what happens to "us" after we die became a spiritual quest. I needed to understand why my beautiful little sister would only get six years on earth. Where did she go? I used to have a sense of being in a body –not being the body – but inhabiting it, and how capricious it was that I landed in the body of a girl, Julia, in the Midwest in a family like mine. We had friends – Catholics – who had 10 kids. I wondered why I didn't end up in that family. Or, once I found out that Michael Jackson's brother Marlon was born on March 12 like me, the same exact year – and in Gary, Indiana, about 30 minutes away from where I was born on Lake Michigan – why didn't I end up as him? Not that I wanted to be someone else, but it felt as if we were all temporary body-temple dwellers.

Nancy had died but something of her stayed close to me, especially right after we lost her. Her energy, her spirit, her love – it stays with me still. As a nine-year-old child I felt this and had no one who could explain to me what was happening – why it happened and what was going to happen. This event completely changed the course of my life in that I became a seeker.

This little cancer warrior lives on in my heart though it's been 55 years. I'll never forget how her sunny, gorgeous personality never dimmed. She never complained about the grueling medical procedures, she lived her life with such love & joy. Always singing, always happy, flashing her dark sparkling eyes in a tiny face. ANGELIC beauty inside & out.

My dad gathered his other three girls in his arms the day she died and said, "Always see her growing up in your mind." Every year her birthday rolls around, she becomes more beautiful and older as we have aged together in my heart and being.

Pediatric oncology was in the dark ages just like juvenile diabetes care was in the 1960s. Doctors would do anything to save the life of a child, even if clearly terminal. Now, we know palliative care at home, with hospice support, is the most desirable way to assist anyone who is terminal.

We celebrate fitness and our bodies when they're vibrantly healthy, toned, and strong. I also celebrate and support those who have another task with their bodies – to survive breast cancer or some other disease.

I've walked on both sides of the street – near death and with vibrant health.

They are flip sides of the same coin, because we can never get away from being in a body. (Until death do us part!)

We can make the "body experience" the best it can be through self-care, self-love and any level of commitment to fitness & nutrition.

I see myself as Soul – not a body with a soul, but a soul with a body. At night in my dreams, I feel myself coming and going to places that are on invisible planes to our physical eyes but I feel them inside in my waking hours. It makes this life seem like the dream, as it can be so real in the dream. Lucid is not a strong enough word.

When I have faced my own mortality and come close to dying myself, or thought my days were going to be short and few, there was a sense of a group of Souls waiting for me on that invisible side. We are deeply connected by love bonds that say: everything will be okay. We're waiting for you when you are ready, we're here. No hurry.

I believe this life is for learning spiritual lessons, for giving love and receiving love. If there was no resistance to what we need to learn, then what would we learn? I got the exact perfect mother I needed – in fact I think we had an agreement – that we choose our parents and they agree to shepherd us into the world, and give us what we need. It may not be what we think we need – as in my case. I needed love in a way that was specific to who I was but got it in a different way and it caused me to grow and stretch as a human being. It gave me strength and a strong sense of what I *did* need. So, the hardships become the gifts.

I always felt connected to a Divine Source within myself. It was a Presence I had always felt as a young child – too big for my mind to hold long. God was no longer a robed, bearded white man in sandals who lived in the clouds. That was only in my imagination.

This Divine Source was a pure loving energy – and not only did it surround me but I felt connected and part of it. It did not line up with the religious tradition in which I was raised. That was part of the appeal, as I had given up on ever understanding through that tradition why I was here and who I was. I felt like I had landed on an alien planet, and my true identity was a secret – even to myself.

I began to explore other sacred teachings at age 17 – many from Eastern roots – and discovered a spiritual practice of chanting sacred words for upliftment. I read Kahil Gibran,

Rumi, Buddhist texts, the Bhagavad Gita, Egyptian Book of the Dead. I read about the Rosicrucians, Edgar Cayce and Madame Blavatsky. I was searching for the answers to life and death – what it all meant.

A friend told me about HU – an ancient name and mantra for the Divine, but also the sound of life itself – if God's love had a sound, it would be HUUUUUUUU. I learned to sing this word softly with attention on my third eye – that point between the brows – where our mind screen is. HU is not specific to any religion, faith, or teaching. I learned it had been in existence for centuries in all parts of the world. Many ancient cultures knew of it and used it for spiritual upliftment.

When I chanted, or sang HU, this ancient mantra relaxed and calmed me, opened me to spiritual ideas I never had before. It was like opening a secret box that spilled out jewels of wisdom that did not come from me, but through me. The possibility of miracles, the way thoughts manifest our reality, how we have total power to change our lives. I was just learning all of this, and in addition: ways to heal myself.

Healing has been a theme my entire life. Healing from loss, grief, and physical and emotional ailments. After being diabetic for six years, the thought of a spiritual healing seemed possible. I didn't know how. But the idea — that it *was* possible — came into my mind like a soft announcement.

I decided to fervently pray to God and ask for a spiritual healing from diabetes. By age 17 I had struggled with infections, high and low blood sugars, vision problems, digestive and nerve damage problems. I was hospitalized so many times, as the diabetes affected my ability to heal quickly from infections. As a young teen, I had to bring my syringes and insulin, which had to be refrigerated, everywhere I went. No matter what I did, there were more days than not that I felt absolutely sick.

15

At age 17, on a summer night, I was sitting up on my bed in the dark. It was the same bedroom where I pleaded with Jesus to make an appearance or give me a sign that he was real.

I looked out at the same dark backyard that ended at the ravine with trees in full leaf. The night crickets were chirping. It brought back a time when I experienced the magical in life. When I saw things in splendor and wonder. I was three, on the back porch on a similar summer night listening to the crickets, when I turned to my parents and said: "Listen! The bunnies are clapping their hands!"

The wonder and magic of life had been clouded by the loss of my sister, the development of diabetes, and my daily struggle as a diabetic. I still had hope things could get better. That I could be healed of diabetes.

This night I made the most heartfelt prayer to God. A huge divine Presence enveloped me and made me feel that life had a purpose. That I had a purpose. I sincerely asked to be healed of diabetes. It was such a brutal disease. There were days I dreaded having to manage it every moment. On a deep level I knew a healing was possible. Somehow. Somehow. It was possible.

To my surprise, a message came gently into my consciousness. A full-on feeling of communication and acknowledgement of my prayer. An answer!

"You will be healed of diabetes."

I didn't feel emotional — just total PEACE. I'd been heard. The diabetes dread disappeared. I reveled in the feeling of not having diabetes. My next thought was:

"But, how?" I asked.

"You will wake up one morning and the diabetes will be gone."

I WILL WAKE UP ONE MORNING AND THE DIABETES WILL BE GONE.

It was like a secret between me and God. That Divine presence said I would be healed of diabetes. I trusted this with all I had. No doubts. I didn't breathe a word of it to anyone. Who would I tell? I have learned that this kind of communication is not for others, and I only share it now because it's been years and was a significantly profound experience. It was deeply, deeply personal and gave me such PEACE.

For the first few months after this, I would awaken in the mornings and wonder, is this the day? Will I know when I don't have to take insulin anymore? Will I have to confirm it with the doctor? Will my blood sugar readings stabilize when I stop taking the insulin? I wonder how I will know. *You'll wake up one morning and the diabetes will be gone* kept coming into my consciousness. I was believing in the magic of life again, that cricket sounds really are bunnies clapping their hands in twilight forests.

But the months passed and then the years. Instead of getting better, I got worse. There were hospitalizations, infections, a near-death experience from septic shock. And then finally a full decade later, at age 27, my kidneys began to fail. Frankly, I had forgotten about the promised healing. It had given me the peace I sought — but not the healing.

Maybe the PEACE was the HEALING.

I got on with my life.

I did the best I could, learning as much as possible about new research in diabetes care. I learned compassion for others who were diseased, disabled, or unwell. I learned to read my body, listen to its intelligence, and be in touch with every aspect of its care and symptoms – and what I had to do for optimal wellness.

At age 17 as a diabetic, I didn't know what I would be facing in the future. It was exactly 17 years later that I would find out.

REFLECTIONS

My body seemed dispensable and capricious in the way it existed in the world. My sister died, I got diabetes, baby brothers came into the world. Looking out at the world from young eyes that only search for love, we might have been rejected, or not getting the kind of love we need. We began to believe we don't deserve it.

My emotionally absent mother denied her deepest feelings in the face of grief and shut herself behind the Bible, OCD organization of house and home as well as church office, and did not value herself. No one taught her to.

When unwarranted parental anger and frustration are projected onto our sensitive beings as children, we take that to mean we are pretty worthless. Our mothers do their best in the face of whatever life hands them. For my mom it was the most extreme punch in life ever – losing a child.

I left the tribe early to find what I was searching for, which was inside me all the time. We don't know that as children. That's the mortal journey leading us to the mystical journey of ourselves.

Our body is the battle field in these advanced courses of "know thyself," which do not come without hardship. On-my-knees-on-the-ground hardship.

The diabetes ravaged my young physical body while my emotions and mental perspective ravaged the rest of me. Meanwhile, I, as an observant Soul, or my higher self – just watched.

Have you ever experienced this part of yourself? The part with the overview – detached from the chains of imprisonment and life stuck-ness. (The part that knew I had diabetes before my father announced it post doctor phone call.)

See this part of you observe your thoughts as if from a bridge spanning a stream that is always moving. Your perspective is looking over the edge of the bridge watching the flow of thoughts, like water, pass beneath and move on.

Learn that what you throw in that river stream either pollutes it or keeps it pure. We are usually really good at throwing junk in there. Junk in, junk out: life can be a knotted mess of low self-esteem expressed and reflected in our treatment of body, emotions, and thought processes.

TO JOURNAL

- List three things you would lovingly tell your younger self about life that you didn't know back then.
- How do you show compassion and love to others? How can you extend that compassion to yourself?
- Who do you most trust? Why?
- What junk can you let go of and not throw in your thought stream?
- What can you put into your thought stream to purify and uplift your everyday life?

TWO

THERE IS NO MAGIC DRAGON NAMED PUFF

People think taking insulin is a cure for diabetes. It's simply a Band-Aid, though. Before the discovery of insulin by Dr. Frederick Banting and Dr. Charles Best in early 1920, patients could be made to live longer by avoiding all carbohydrates, living on protein and fats. To live a year or two with Type 1 diabetes was exceptional, as the body would go into ketoacidosis and begin feeding on itself for fuel. The bloodstream would become toxic as the person wasted away on the fainting couch or in bed. Children would be in a diabetic coma, grieving parents making funeral arrangements. There is a photo from 1922 of a ward of children all in comatose diabetic ketoacidosis. Scientists entered and began injecting the children with a new drug – insulin, Before they had injected the last child, the first woke up. One by one all the children came out of the diabetic coma. A room full of death became one of joy and hope.*

---

* https://diabeteshopefoundation.com/

A mild ketogenic state is now a strategy for losing weight. I cannot think of a more unappetizing way to "get skinny." It's not the same as ketoacidosis, of course. And like many, I have tried it, but became very sick in my 40's at the same time. It's hard on the kidneys.

My case of juvenile Type 1 diabetes was labile - hard to control and brittle. This is not the case for all. I have known diabetics in their 50s diagnosed at age two — who have had no complications. For those of us who have, however, it's a slow death — as uncontrolled blood sugars and high glucose levels in the blood continue to erode the vascular and nervous system of the body. This is what leads to blindness, kidney failure, heart disease, amputations, and nerve damage.

In the 1960's diabetes was considered "an old person's disease." Everyone had a grandparent who had diabetes, had gone blind, lost a few toes to amputation or even a foot or leg. It was a terrible disease to get in old age but since the person was old anyway not much research was done to investigate better care.

Enter juvenile onset diabetes — or Type 1. I'm not talking about Type 2, which is the domain of the "over forty and overweight." In children, research has shown it's brought on by an autoimmune response. And the cause of that response in the most current research is what is called a Serious Life Event (SLE.) For me that was obvious — my sister's death, compounded by an emotionally absent mother and no opportunity to grieve deeply about the loss of my little sister, Nancy. Other events took place in my pre-teen life that eroded my sense of the world being a safe place. I learned not to let down my guard and keep a happy face outwardly to the world. I wasn't going to cave on any level. Or show weakness.

After I was out of the hospital and got home, life again took on a rhythm. I was 12 and it didn't seem to affect my sports activity at school. I took orange juice to the nurse's station at school every week in case of a hypoglycemic episode. Mixed with a tablespoon of sugar, it would bring my blood sugar back up, but always overshoot the mark and be very high for the next 24 hours. I couldn't seem to win the balancing act. No one explained to me that this was not normal for a diabetic. The sporadic doctor's visits were useless, so I just got on with it the best I could.

My menses started at age 14 – and with it came a voracious appetite and craving for sweets and carbs. At our house there were always potato chips, cookies, canned nuts, and homemade desserts. The pantry was filled with junk food: Ding Dongs, Twinkies, and Oreos. Even though my mother was health conscious, took vitamins and swam every day and in her later years at 85, walked two miles a day, there were sweets around all the time. At 14 I would get home from school at 4 p.m. and be starving. I could eat a family size bag of barbecued potato chips in one sitting of the soap opera on TV, "Dark Shadows."

Seemingly overnight, I gained weight and my clothes got tight. I didn't like the feeling. My mother began to make comments about my body and how it was not what it should be. I felt her disapproval in my appearance. She made an appointment with a diabetic specialist, a doctor my parents were friends with from their country club. The visits were always the same. A social time that was worthless to my concerns and state of my body as a young diabetic. I never learned anything new, was not told how to make things better, or given any feedback for what I did right. After a blood test, they would mostly talk about social topics, people and golf. I didn't feel I was there for any reason other than for them to visit.

I'd be given a stick to pass through a stream of my urine and if it turned purple – that was bad – it meant my blood sugars had been high in the last 12 hours (but maybe not now) and my body was excreting sugar and ketones through urination. If it didn't change color, I was not spilling sugar or ketones in my urine. But the urine was hours old and not relative to the moment. It was so inaccurate. You could not play catch-up with insulin, which took time to act, and I only took one shot a day. It was the best they had at the time. A full blood draw was the only way to get an accurate, real-time blood-sugar reading and that happened only at the doctor's office.

The doctor understood that I had started my period and developed a runaway appetite. It was causing me distress. He took out a prescription pad and scribbled on it, handed the prescription to my mom and said, "This medication can help with your appetite. Take two a day." We went to the pharmacy. I saw they were little white pills. They were Benzedrine, also called "Bennies," which were a popular street drug, I was to learn later in life. They were to help me lose weight.

After four days of taking Benzedrine, I was jittery and anxious. I didn't like it at all. I stopped taking the pills. Giving speed to a 14-year-old who wants to lose weight? Medicine was just so wrong back then. Part of my medical journey has been to see how things have changed over the decades – how research and clinical case studies inform newly minted doctors. How patients demand certain services from their health care teams – such as compassionate care, partnering on treatment decision-making, and questioning advice. You always need an advocate! A loved one who can make decisions if you are not able to. Or demand better nursing care in the hospital if you are too weak from surgery to ask for what you need. Most of all, I've learned doctors are not infallible and it's okay to challenge their opinions. Such as: you will never get back to the weight you were in your 20's. Or, this medication will cause you to gain 30 or 40 pounds. Or this medication will help you lose weight – and ratchet your anxiety levels off the chart.

So, at 14, I continued to gain weight and struggle with diabetes. It all felt so out of my control. No adults to talk to or understand what it was like to constantly monitor normal things like eating and exercising (which I didn't do much of beyond cheerleading, swimming, and track seasonally.) All of this stress in my early teens found an outlet in me — experimenting with recreational drugs. I would forget to eat; I began to lose weight. It was not an ideal situation – but one in a long line of experiences where I wanted my body to be one way, but it was another. I was a risk taker who often felt, what do I have to lose? It's better than staying in one place getting nowhere.

When I went away to boarding school at age 16, 2,000 miles away from home, I had an epiphany that followed a very traumatic drug experience: I alone was responsible for all that happened to me – especially the bad, because I'd allowed it.

Being away from the family environment (at my request – my parents actually allowed this) for my junior and senior years of high school, I was handed a level of freedom I never had before. Without any wisdom, a low level of self-esteem and loathing my body, I willingly ingested dangerous street drugs without forethought. The epiphany came right on the heels of an extremely traumatic drug experience using LSD I will never forget – or want to repeat. I was disconnected from all reality during this experience. I had chosen to be by myself before the LSD took effect. Once it kicked in, I lost myself in terrifying sights and sounds that didn't exist.

I will describe this experience later, but because of it, I let go of recreational drugs. I could not risk my sanity, and it had been taken from me for a few hours in a snowy field on a winter's day when I was all alone.

I found other outlets to soothe my restlessness and the longing for meaning in life I was seeking. I loved nature and found peace in the forests and lakes that bordered the school campus. I got more involved in making art of all kinds during the long New England winters. I was hiking, mountain climbing, rappelling. It was naturally slimming me down and I was eating carefully, weighing my food and taking care of myself. I began to feel better than I had in years – with energy and a level blood sugar – and that brought home the erratic health situation I had accepted in taking risks in my life choices. I was 16 years old and I realized the diabetes had no steward but me. If I wanted to feel better, I had to follow the protocol that was advised about food. Prepare for low blood-sugar episodes, watch out for infections, rest when I needed to. I had advocates — the school cook and the school nurse became my surrogate moms. They looked out for me, and made sure I was on track. It was more than I had gotten in my family home. As an adult I understand the circumstances of why this was. My parents were essentially raising a second family with my younger sister and two baby brothers. My older sister and I – our needs were secondary if considered at all. I was beginning to take care of myself like an adult at age 16.

A behavior I learned as a child: if I got sick, I'd get the love and attention I needed from my mother. She was very proficient at the mother role – birthday parties, holidays, day-to-day care of us kids. From my perspective, though, it was without joy. It was a sense of duty and often exasperated her, tired her out, and lacked any love. She was not a touchy-feely person; I honestly don't remember getting hugs from her. My dad was the affectionate one. I felt a closeness to him my entire life – from early childhood on we had a special bond. He was approachable and gentle, accepting and supportive emotionally to all his kids. His day was spent with the family business and he didn't see my mother's anger like we did. If my parents argued, we never heard it. Later I was angry with my dad for not protecting me from my mother's rages but what I learned from him was to keep my focus forward, think positively and always, always, do the right thing.

Being a feeling, sensitive child seemed to make me a target for my mother's anger. If she felt powerless, seeing me react emotionally to her anger must have given her some sense of dominion over her world. It caused me to be my own care-taker. I put on armor emotionally and I didn't trust her. This pushed me outside the safety of the tribe of my family, while I was very young. First emotionally, then physically in my mid-teens, when I begged to be sent to a boarding school. This self-reliance made me a strong person. It was the gift and result of having a mother like mine. She was one of my best "spiritual" teachers.

When I was seven, the doctors found a blood clot in my right eye that needed to be surgically removed. My mother and I traveled to Chicago for the best surgeon. It was just the two of us who took the train from my grandmother's house into the city. It felt like an adventure. She was attentive and fun on the ride. A young man with a guitar saw me, came over and sang *Puff the Magic Dragon*.

If getting sick or having an illness brought this much love, attention and fun, well . . . maybe I should get sick more often?

Puff the magic dragon lived by the sea
And frolicked in the autumn mist in a land called Honah Lee
Little Jackie Paper loved that rascal Puff
And brought him strings and sealing wax and other fancy stuff

Oh, Puff the magic dragon lived by the sea
And frolicked in the autumn mist in a land called Honah Lee
Puff the magic dragon lived by the sea
And frolicked in the autumn mist in a land called Honah Lee

Together they would travel on a boat with billowed sail
Jackie kept a lookout perched on Puff's gigantic tail
Noble kings and princes would bow whene'er they came
Pirate ships would lower their flags when Puff roared out his name

After the operation, I spent several nights in the hospital on white starched, scratchy hospital sheets that smelled like disinfectant. I had a small hospital gown, and they gave me underwear. Though clean, they had fecal stains from other small patients, and I didn't want to wear them. When I could get out of bed, and the eye patch was off, I went to the bathroom mirror and looked at my eye. It was red and swollen but the operation was a success. It was my first time having surgery. I was also the first of four children to have any medical issues. Nancy had not gotten sick yet. The following year, she would.

We took the train back to my grandmother's and then drove home. My mom pulled into our driveway. I got out of the car. It had been a fun adventure despite waking up with a patched eye and feeling pain and grogginess. I got sung to on the train by a man.

As I stood in the driveway, my mother's mood changed. I remember feeling so let down when she fell back into her angry, temperamental, unloving self. Something about the pressures of being home must have triggered her impatience and angry mood. I thought it was me. I was the bad child. I felt a weight settle on my shoulders again. Life seemed to just go up and down that way.

Growing up, I experienced bright spots. Every summer, we spent the entire day at the country-club pool. It was on the other side of town and built on top of a hill, surrounded by green rolling hills and gullies. There was a golf course designed around it. My dad won many championships there, and was a great friend with the golf pro in the shop as well as the restaurant and bar staff. Everyone seemed to know and love my dad. My mom fit the perfect example of a 60's housewife with four little girls, a pretty lady with a ready smile. I wished she would be like that at home.

The pool was on the top of the highest hill and had a nearby snack bar. We'd start swim-team practice at 7:30 a.m. and stay until 5 p.m. My mother would simply drop us off and come back at 5. The swim-team coaches knew all the kids and so did the lifeguards. As a membership-only club, it was a perfectly safe place to be.

The snack bar offered the smell of burgers and French fries. Anytime we were hungry we'd go into the snack bar, order and put it on Dad's bill, including popsicles and ice cream bars. My body was tanned and brown, and my arms were hard from swim-team practice. I felt strong. The golf course surrounding the pool up on the hill allowed us to look down from the high dive and see golfers teeing off. The bright green fairways curled around huge, old-growth trees and sand traps; cicadas sang in waves of sound. I was a water baby and loved to swim. Those were idyllic days.

I became aware of my body as well as the bodies of other females. There were several women in their 40's and 50's who were in bikinis, smoking cigarettes by the pool. They looked chic, tan and relaxed, but as I think back, not healthy. They were so skinny – and later I found out that the same doctor treating my diabetes was also dispensing Benzedrine to these women for weight loss. The cigarettes helped, too. They were the Midwest version of the "ladies who lunch" but laid by the pool and skipped lunch.

There were the girls in high school who looked like the model Twiggy. I could see their jutting hip bones and bony shoulders – their flat bellies, stick arms and legs, sunken cheeks and eyes – I heard the word anorexia. Their bikinis barely held on.

My own body was not changing fast enough for me – I would stand in front of the mirror and wonder if I would ever get boobs. I was strong, athletic and fit, but at this point I was learning to find things about my body I didn't like. Besides the diabetes and having no control over my blood-sugar swings at times, I also hated the way I looked. I didn't care if boys thought I was cute, I didn't feel that way.

These ingrained ideas come upon us as vulnerable children and just because we THINK it, we believe it's true. So many of these ideas settled within my being from an early age – we all have them – and they sabotage us later. Somewhere deep down, we don't feel worthy, or loveable, or attractive. Or we are accused of being selfish, too sensitive, or when genuine emotion is being expressed, we are "putting on an act." I was so unconscious of these limiting ideas until I got into relationships with men later in life that reinforced the subconscious ideas, I carried deep inside me: thoughts of being unworthy, undeserving, unlovable. My body became the battlefield for such limiting ideas in how cavalierly I treated it. I had cycles of caring for my health and body, but it was the first thing to suffer when I was going through a rough emotional time. It would manifest as binge eating. Food seemed to help "stuff" my feelings.

REFLECTIONS

Our toxic relationship with food can reflect our toxic relationships with ourselves — and in my case, with men. Until I was 28, I chose the "bad boys." Unknowingly, I was choosing the ones who reinforced my low self-esteem. I piled on by punishing myself with food — unconscious eating, emotional eating. I had buried feelings, and food stuffed them further down.

A first marriage that lasted only 10 months changed things dramatically. I call that my "practice husband" because I had to change who I was attracting into my life.

I had to change ME.

Low self-esteem can be buried so deep we aren't even aware of it. Outwardly we may look successful, but buried false beliefs about self often surface when we try to change our lives, our perspective, or tackle getting healthy and fit once and for all.

Facing oneself takes work and courage.

Every relationship we have reflects our relationship with ourselves. An offshoot of that is our relationship with food. It becomes a punishing activity, based in self-hate but we have no idea how that started. However, it can end with self-love being practiced daily. Love your body as it is now. Stop when you feel you are weaponizing food against yourself and ask why. What is behind this behavior? True transformation starts with the relationship with yourself.

You deserve love, abundance, success, and your wildest dreams. A healthy body (through your own efforts) is proof you believe it and are rocking self-love.

You are a series of invisible wheels with one visible wheel: your body. The three other wheels seem invisible at times. We often hear body – mind – spirit – but I recognize body – emotions – mind – spirit.

Your mind acts like a computer – generating thoughts that start in the emotions and the body – and what a wild ride of thoughts maybe you've had over the tempo of time. Your spirit (your real identity seems to watch from afar but drives the chariot) just observes as these wheels turn and turn. To get them to turn in tandem is the greatest challenge. Mind pushes emotions, emotions push the body, the body pushes mind. When I say "push" I mean that those wheels are turned up high and caused this kind of overflow of energy that was seeking balance. It often manifests in negative body image, unconscious eating, bingeing, and a feeling of being out of control.

When you start weight lifting and training, learning more about nutrition, there is a day- in-and-day-out rhythm that completely envelopes those turning wheels. Over time (give it a year or more!) they began to spin in tandem, in balance, and with positive results in your mind, emotions, and body. It flows like a river and has its own timing.

TO JOURNAL

- Does your relationship with food reflect your relationship with yourself?
- What ambitions do you have for your health to increase your enjoyment of daily living?
- Are you aware of a part of you that watches yourself thinking?
- What mental habits are habitual but no longer serve you?
- How might you change one habit that no longer serves you with a habit that is completely goal-directed? Goal example: Improve health and wellness.

THREE

SNOW QUEEN

When I was in fifth grade there was a ridiculous contest that exacerbated the already cruel tendencies of pre-teen girls. There is no meaner bully than a female 12-13-year-old. She is just beginning to feel her power and very often it's turned up high in the form of abuse of the girls around her.

My sister had died when I was 9 – and now I was 11 – two years since that Serious Life Event. At the elementary school I attended the traditional popularity contest of SNOW QUEEN was taking place in December. The winning girl got to ride in the Christmas parade in an open Corvette (despite the cold) waving to the crowd as the most popular girl representing her school. Who thought this contest up? It had been happening for years.

One of my friends had an older sister who won Snow Queen two years before. I'll call her Jane. Jane was determined to catch the same title at any expense. Frankly I was her biggest competition. We were in the "popular girls" clique and I had a sense of this but didn't gloat about it – we were just a circle of friends who knew each other for years. We were all active and engaged in sports, went to the same slumber parties, our parents belonged to the same country club, we were on swim team together. This pulled us together more than being popular.

Another girl I'll call Lisa, was my very best friend from first grade. She lived nearby, across the ravine behind our house, and we walked to school together every day for years. Lisa was the bestie of besties. We took her on our family vacations to Florida, and I went with her family on theirs. We hung out every weekend, went to the skating rink, movies, bowling, and birthday parties together. We were cheerleaders together. We did our first slow dance with Kent and Frank when we were 13, one summer day at her house when her parents weren't home. I'll never forget the greenness of the trees out the window of her ultra-modern glass house swaying to some pop 40 ballad hugging Kent. We talked about boys, shared secrets and intertwined our lives for many years.

But the Snow Queen contest loomed and Jane, determined to win, used a strategy that to this day baffles me – how she got it to work. What did she say, do, or create to make this situation work in her favor.

It was two weeks before the voting took place. Suddenly my bestie of besties, Lisa, found excuses not to walk to school with me or could not hang out on the weekends. At first, I was confused but then she told me her mother didn't want her to associate with me anymore. I was dumbfounded and very hurt. I didn't tell anyone. I felt so ashamed. Why would her mother suddenly not like me? I had gone to Florida with them the previous year on vacation. What did I do so that her mother didn't like me at all now and forbade Lisa to spend time with me? I was humiliated.

Then things at school got worse. The rest of my circle of friends began to move away from me – literally — if I came down the school hallway. No one would sit with me in class or on the playground. No one would talk to me. I wasn't invited to parties. I was shunned by this circle of friends. Worst of all, my bestie, Lisa, had joined in. There was more shame and humiliation. I blamed myself somehow. I was 11 years old.

We lived close to the elementary school so I walked home for lunch every day. It was the day one of the girls faked a coughing fit when I walked by in the hall that broke me. Two friends giggled and joined in like I was some walking disease.

I left for lunch and walked home with tears in my eyes. Devastated, confused, humiliated, and ashamed, I had no idea what was going on. I burst into the house sobbing. My mother was setting lunch out for us three girls and feeding the baby in his high chair.

"What's wrong?!" There was annoyance in her voice. I told her all my friends at school were ignoring me and that Lisa would not even walk to school with me anymore. I couldn't explain beyond that. Like how long it had been going on, that Lisa's mother hated me now, and I wasn't invited to parties. I couldn't because I was sobbing uncontrollably.

My mother continued to make lunch and looked up for a moment. Bobby was in his high chair eating Spaghetti-Os.

"It must have been something you did!" she said accusingly, and turned back to the food on the counter.

That was December, 1968. Two months later I was in the hospital diagnosed with juvenile onset Type 1 diabetes. I believe this experience contributed to my onset of diabetes as an autoimmune response to stress that had started with my sister dying, my mother shutting down emotionally, my friends shunning and bullying me. This was the final blow.

Jane did win Snow Queen and so carried on the shallow tradition in her family that seemed so important to her. I no longer considered these girls my friends, and moved away from that circle. It took years but Lisa came around again. She had been a weak pawn in the face of such bullying tactics. Ultimately, she abandoned our friendship again after college. She never gave a reason. But we certainly grew apart.

I have seen how women treat each other and I wish we could lift each other up and be kind. We are all sensitive creatures – men too – and women have a propensity to give their all. And to feel guilty and to not feel beautiful enough, worthy enough, thin enough, simply not enough of anything that society puts on us. Sometimes we are raised by women who do not know their worth because of the times, society's expectations, or family dysfunction of their own in child-hood. The low self-esteem is passed on. We don't learn to value ourselves and to love who we are.

Coupled with family dynamics of growing up and experiences we have as children, it can turn into a huge mess: a lack of confidence, lack of self-worth, no self-acceptance and no self-love. I was ashamed of whatever it was in me that caused that circle of friends to abandon me. I thought it was my fault. My mother confirmed my fear with her offhanded comment just when I needed reassurance the most.

My sister's death carried with it an exploding bomb that affected the entire family. My mother was at ground zero for most of the year that Nancy suffered the indignities of pediatric cancer care – there was no palliative care back then and doctors went beyond where they should to save the life of a child who was terminal. The child suffered, the parents suffered, the siblings suffered.

My mother did the absolute best she could, but I just can't imagine what this did to her heart and soul. She was already angry before Nancy's diagnosis. Now after her death, she was trying to find peace in religion. When Nancy had her first operation, to remove the tumor in her little abdomen, my mother would heat up pure cocoa butter on the stove to smooth over Nancy's healing incision. The tumor grew back. It was an aggressive sarcoma. In her every move, she devoted herself to Nancy's care. She bore this burden pretty much alone, as my dad was always working. The three other daughters – we had no idea what was really happening to Nancy, just that she was in and out of the hospital and getting thinner each time she came home.

I cannot imagine what my parents experienced losing this beautiful, dark-haired 6-year-old who had no idea she was going to die. Her eyes continued to sparkle with joy, she sang songs in her sweet voice, was a gentle loving child with the apropos middle name of Adore, a combination of our two grandmother's names. Over the course of the year, she wasted away to nothing but skin and bones, with huge, round, trusting brown eyes. When she got pneumonia, she looked at my mother and said,

"When I breathe, something breathes with me."

It was the death of this beloved child that brought my mother into a completely different state. She shut down emotionally. If she was angry before, it became more so. Decades later, she told me how angry she was with God when Nancy died. The pain was still etched in her face, and the grief in her eyes was as if it had just happened. I was in my 50's then. It was the first glimpse of how truly searing the grief continued to be – she never lifted the veil on it ever again.

I read the obituary in the local paper for Nancy when she died in September of 1966. It said she was "survived" by … then named my parents, and us three girls, her sisters. I felt so angry. It was not true. I was not "surviving." I was drowning in pain and grief. They used the wrong word in the paper.

I learned to hate the word "cancer." In my third-grade class a few weeks later, we were learning geography, and the teacher mentioned "the Tropic of Cancer." I wondered how she could be so mean to say that word in front of me? After my sister died of it? My grief was like a hard glass bubble that I lived in, alone. Couldn't everyone see I needed to be reassured, allowed to feel the grief, I needed comfort, I needed love and understanding. Don't say the word "Cancer" when I am around.

For my mother the church became her refuge. The dogma shielded her somehow, but it felt like she was hiding behind a wall. She doubled down on church-going, bible-reading, and pushing us three girls to accept Jesus as savior or go to hell. She felt that was her mission in life as a mother, a newly discovered mission. Before, church felt like a family obligation to show up as a unit. Like when we had to stand in the vestibule, all of us girls with our parents, and greet the church members as they arrived for services. It felt like a charade. The hose I had to wear itched. We wore matching dresses. The perfect family. I felt like it was an act, a performance. Everyone so polite, no one being real.

But now, it was more about salvation, and the mission my mother felt called to complete. I was forced to go to church and believe what she insisted we believe. As if an angry mother telling me I had to go to church would in any way give me spiritual comfort or salvation. My survivor instincts – and I did have them! – kicked in and I rebelled against that kind of brainwashing. I saw the outright hypocrisy through a child's eyes. Compassion and understanding for what my mother endured and hoped for in life did not come to me until I was much older. She was alone in many ways, struggling with all life handed her, and society expected of her.

As a spiritual child, and later a seeker of Truth, my mother's religious views and demands were not something I could accept. I would not be forced to do or believe anything. It became a hallmark of my survival instincts. But I was completely alone in my grief. I walled myself in. I stayed in my glass bubble, alone. Nancy was not talked about after the first few weeks of intense pain and loss. We didn't get any counseling. There was no bereavement support back then. Even though my parents had turned to the pastor of their church for solace, we children were not a part of those meetings at the time.

My sister's death left a wound and a scar on my inner world that caused me to search for life's meaning. Death of a loved one has a way of doing that. When you are a child, it's years and years before you reach any peace. The realness of her absence through death of her body sparked in me a deep desire to know how the invisible side of life worked. I'd had "extra sensory perception" experiences – or ESP – that reached into an invisible reality I could feel but didn't understand. It seemed connected to Nancy and the answers I needed about why she had to die and where she went. I could almost lift the veil and see the beyond, but it was as if I had not earned the strength yet to fully see and fully know.

The beautiful child that was me, was so open, so willing and so vulnerable. I questioned why I was here but *did not know* why I was here. When I look into my inner-child eyes, I love her and want her to know everything will be okay despite what is to come into her life. She is so young. I came here with a purpose and when I was a baby I looked out of those eyes, observed where I was and wondered nothing – just observed. As I grew, I became more interested in this place and knew there was a secret being held from me of why I was here – and then … who was I, really? Who was I and why was I here? I had the overwhelming feeling I was here to do something but what was it?

My family life with its periods of dysfunction and loss made me strong so I could survive this journey – and it was not love (the kind I thought I needed) that I was given on a deep level, it was strife and challenges. It caused me to look within myself for the strength and answers. Anyone who knows my family growing up would not have seen the strife, the pain, the dysfunction. My perception was driven by my own need for love, — given in a certain way and not getting it. It was how I processed the experiences. It gave me grit.

I was a fighter, determined to move forward and keep going no matter what. It's the only thing that has mattered, except my love for the Divine, for God, for understanding my connection to the Life Force that is in everything, that is in me and is me. That has been my stay, my safety, my Amazing Grace. It's a seat of awareness in which I sit to observe my life, not always successfully and as a child not at all. Those were the answers I sought. Even though I felt alone at times, there was not really a deep darkness – there was always that Presence.

The lack of love in my childhood from my mother — as I understood and needed love — was a way for me to go beyond my own family borders, and find a new tribe, and a new way of living that was not constrained. I was a rebel and the pain I felt caused me to take risks as a teenager. It caused my parents added stress to an already difficult family life, of losing a child and adding two more. I honestly love my parents, both now deceased. My mother was a hard one to love and hard to get love from – and my dad was that stable father who was always my cheerleader, very caring, very supportive, able to express his love and his pride.

At age 15 I moved out of the family house in the summer for two weeks with a friend whose parents were much more liberal than mine. I didn't ask my parents, I told them. We rented a room in the house of a single math professor in exchange for cleaning and cooking. Cooking was heating a can of soup on the stove. At night he would bring home prostitutes, but he left us alone.

After two weeks, a knock came at the door of our rental. It was my dad.

"Honey, get your bag. You're coming home."

He looked like he would cry if I said no. I got my bag and we left the math professor's house. The kid who provided us with marijuana, Pancho, had been there in the living room of the rental. My father never forgot the threat he felt at the presence of Pancho. Even in my 40s he mentioned it. It haunted him, and me too, that I put him through such a time.

Things didn't get better. I hated Indiana, and I was so tired of the people I grew up with –how I was identified in a narrow way by my peers, as a popular, bubbly, cheerleader with lots of friends — when in fact inside I was dark and brooding. I wondered what life held for me. Whatever it was I would not find it in my home, my school, my town. I wanted out! I was a sophomore in high school and already dreaded junior year in Indiana.

That year, a friend went to boarding school in California. It felt like a possible escape for me. It sounded like a great idea and I excitedly proposed this to my parents. No one I knew ever went to boarding school – our educational system was so highly rated in our town.

I proposed this to my parents and my father gave it some thought and came up with an idea. He made some calls and suggested sending me to Culver Military Academy, his high school alma mater a few hours' drive away. I absolutely refused to consider such an idea – I was a free spirit, an artist. Military school? NO WAY. We had a shouting match and I ran out of the house to a friend. I felt absolutely trapped. Military school?

Hours later my parents called and said they had an alternative and asked me to come back home. They really did want to find the right answer to my needs, and were willing to consider letting me go away to finish high school at age 16. That they pulled back on the military option was a gift and so was allowing me to go away at all. I had two more years of high school to finish.

They found a clearing house in New York with a list of creative arts' boarding schools. My father suggested we get in the car in August, drive east and visit the ones they had and find the one that was right for me. I was elated. My entire being changed in the next week, knowing I was facing a new life at 16. I was excited to move on – to whatever the future held — and let go of what had become a stagnating existence which I tried to dull with recreational drugs. My parents knew I was experimenting with drugs and their hope was I would get away from that influence.

When my parents finally dropped me off at the creative arts boarding school we decided on, I felt so free. I no longer felt encumbered by the expectations and ideas about my identity after going to school with kids from kindergarten on. I was one of the popular kids. Later in life I realized I had manufactured this outcome in order to feel a part of something where I was liked and accepted because I truly did not feel accepted at home. I felt invisible, despite my closeness with my dad. Once my two brothers were born, all focus was on them and my younger sister. – My older sister and I were forgotten in the hustle and bustle of toddlers over teenagers. I was determined to find my own way and was willing to take risks to change the narrative of my life in my teens.

My parents lived "up the hill" in our Midwest town and my dad was a businessman. My friends were of similar backgrounds. We swam on the same team at the country club, had slumber parties, went to dances and movies, bowled, ice skating rinks in the winter, roller skating rinks in the summer. But they seemed so narrow to me and at 16 I began to make friends with another subgroup in high school who were hippies. They smoked pot and listened to more interesting music than the top 40 radio stations. Their parents lived "down the hill" in the older grand homes that were near

Purdue University. Their parents were artists, photographers, and professors.

I got more involved with this subgroup, and my sense of who I was changed. I had felt locked into a persona that was not really me but that I was labeled. It was a sense of not being seen, not being known or valued either at home or at school by the old crowd. The new crowd felt more alive, accepting and open to more of life's adventures. But it was still Indiana.

My parents and I packed up the car in August, 1973 and drove East. I felt hopeful. Less resentful. Less angry. Excited. When we got into the mountains of Western Massachusetts, we stopped at a cabin along a mountain stream for sandwiches. I was actually enjoying being with my parents.

The first boarding school we visited was Stockbridge School. It was on a beautiful piece of land in the Berkshire Mountains. The main building was the original mansion of the Hannah family – Hannah House — the girl's dorm. There were boys' dorms, a dining hall, art studios, soccer field, and class rooms on this huge acreage. It was tucked against the foothills of the Berkshires and surrounded by forest, foothills, and small lakes.

Arriving, we drove down a wooded country road. A huge green field opened up on a hill to the left with a four-story Gilded Age white clapboard mansion on the top. My eyes followed the mansion as we drove past a long black-iron fence to the main gate.

Stockbridge School.

As soon as we pulled past the huge ornate gate, and up the winding drive, I felt at home. There was a magical energy to the mountains, the old mansion, the campus dotted with old-growth trees.

It was clear to me this was the place when we met the headmaster, Dick Nurse, and his wife, Laura. They wore full Afros and matching Dashikis and I thought they were about the coolest pair of people I had ever seen in my life.

The art teacher, John, was from the UK, the soccer coach, Omar, was from Senegal, and David Gunn, an older African American gentleman, was the physical ed director. Norman Rockwell lived in the nearby town of West Stockbridge. His painting, "The Problem We All Live With" (1964, oil on canvas) was based on little Ruby Bridges being escorted to a desegregated school by four U.S. Marshals. Mr. Rockwell used local models. Coach Gunn's daughter, Lynda, and her cousin Anita, were used as the models for Ruby Bridges – as she was being escorted to school in her beautiful white dress.

The social studies teacher was Yale-educated and looked like Paul Bunyan with a full beard, and a braid all the way down his back. Hippies.

"I want to go here," I announced.

After we met with Dick and Laura Nurse, we went to an outdoor picnic table to talk. The school was founded by Hans Maeder in 1949. He felt teaching tolerance across cultures was not enough. You needed understanding.

From his obituary in the New York Times, September 11, 1988:

> *Mr. Maeder's nonprofit school, Stockbridge, which he and his wife, Ruth, opened in 1949 in Interlaken, Mass., was long considered one of the more progressive private boarding schools in New England in an era when such institutions catered mostly to the children of well-to-do white families.*
>
> *Stockbridge, Mr. Maeder declared, would be interracial, nondenominational and international in outlook, ideals that he said had been inspired by the United Nations Charter. The school dramatized its commitment by flying the United Nations flag just below the American flag. The curriculum included a junior year abroad, and for several years, Stockbridge operated a branch in Corcelles, Switzerland.*
>
> *https://www.nytimes.com/1988/09/11/obituaries/hans-k-maeder-stockbridge-founder-dies-at-78.html*

When I arrived in 1973, Stockbridge had declining fortunes. Mr. Maeder had retired, but the spirit of the place was intact. I went to school with Park Avenue trust funders as well as kids from New York City projects. And the in-betweens like me, a middle-class kid from the Midwest.

Dad gave me a talk about how small the campus would seem at times and to call them anytime if I wanted to come home or it didn't work out – but I was happy to see them go. My mom said she cried all the way home – it was probably a relief I was out of the house. We had been in a difficult relationship for years. Once I was at Stockbridge, months would go by without a word from them – no letters or phone calls. I felt completely forgotten. I know they were consumed with the three younger siblings and getting my older sister ready for college. But me - out of sight, out of mind.

My parents drove off that day and it was the first time I was in a new environment where I didn't know anyone. I felt confident in my ability to make friends and took my time to get to know people. I came from a situation where everyone knew me (or thought they did) and I had lots of friends and admirers. Now I was in a place where no one knew me and no one cared. It was freeing. I could reinvent myself. I was 16 and had this sense I could be exactly who I wanted to be – not made up, but my authentic self without social pressure or preconceived ideas of who I was.

The liberal atmosphere and lack of authority on campus opened a door to freedom I was not prepared to handle well, especially at age 16. The first day I arrived, I went for a walk and got to the edge of the forest. I could see a trail disappearing into the woods. As I stood there looking at the trail, a naked boy of about 17 came around a tree. He had curly wild hair, pimples and a look of utter shock on his face. His eyes were wide, not with fear but with something else. He was muttering, not making sense and he was buck-naked. It turned out he was tripping on LSD.

I made new friends who came from all walks of life, were different races, skin tones, and cultures. I had grown up in an all-white, middle-class world – my parents' closest friends had last names like Cohen, Pearlstein, and Levinson. My Christian parents never pointed out that their friends were Jewish and believed differently than Christians. It was never mentioned.

When I got to Stockbridge School, there were a lot of kids who were Jewish – and proud of it. I got to know an entire culture through them – and wondered why Jews had been so on the down-low in Indiana. Maybe because the KKK had been active in Indiana since 1915. And until the late 60's, Jews were not allowed to join the country club in town.

My new classmates were Dominican, Puerto Rican, Black, Jewish, and plain old White Anglo Saxon Protestant, like me — a WASP.

To this day so many of these classmates who became friends are still my dear friends. Our lives reflect the varying backgrounds we come from but we all love and accept each other as if a day has not passed since Stockbridge School. It was a rare experience that continued to shape my life. But of all my new friends, there was one who would impact my life very deeply. It was meeting Louis that changed my life forever.

REFLECTIONS

Despite the departure from my family home, I took all of my issues with me to my new environment at boarding school. I was indeed happier, glad to be away, but places don't cure our unhappiness, because unhappiness is inside and goes where we go.

A new city, a new partner, a new job, a new body through weight loss or plastic surgery – none of these things hold the key to what we are truly looking for. It's looking from the outside in, not from the inside out.

Your body is connected to your mind and your spirit in an endless loop of energy exchange. We have so much power and control over how our life can go, but we don't use it.

Here's a tip: IMAGINATION.

That's reaching into the deepest part of yourself and creating your life – from thought energy – from imagination – keeping that vision of what you want. Not what you don't want!

Albert Einstein said this – what a modern-day mystic he was!

"Imagination is everything. It is the preview of life's coming attractions."

You imagine something, fill it with positive emotional feeling, believe it deep down, and it will come to pass.

Worry is a toxic form of imagining. Projecting scenarios filled with negative emotion is also a recipe for manifestation. It works no matter if we use it consciously or not.

When we work with positive visioning, the illusion of time throws us off, because things take time to manifest into form. But hang in there, because it's on the way! You have to make a space for it by thinking about it, being dedicated to it, feeling it, living it, being it, and taking steps so it can come into your life.

Fitness is the perfect thing to experiment with to see how this law of manifestation works. But don't fight with yourself and self-sabotage. Like all things, when you do it with LOVE, it works like a dream. A good dream.

Body, mind, and spirit are connected, but we are used to only taking on the body. We forget the two other more important parts.

Your body becomes the form created from the blueprint of your thoughts. It's so important to love your body no matter where you are in your health journey. The body is a magnificent teacher. Fitness is an incredible practice, when you address all three levels: body, mindset, and spirit. This is where true TRANSFORMATION happens, on the inside and in the endless loop of energy we project out here.

TO JOURNAL

- What three conditions or qualities do you want most in your life right now?
- Do you see yourself as successful in achieving these in your life? Why or why not?
- List three small things you can start doing today to move forward in manifesting those three qualities or conditions.

FOUR

LOUIS IN THE SKY WITH DIAMONDS

He was a Jewish kid from New Jersey who proudly sang in Hebrew what he learned during his bar mitzvah. He could charm anyone. He had thick, long, wavy brown hair, expressive, soft brown eyes, and large hands. His nose was one long bone down his face that gave him a noble look – which was quickly ruined by goofy antics. His eyes had a sleepy look and he had a way of chortling that signaled how much he was touched by something. He had a heart like no one I had ever met, and wore it on his sleeve. He chose the most outcast kids on campus to befriend. He didn't like to see anyone left out.

He liked to sing and any circumstance would invite a comment that was sung. If I was making something to eat, it was Hank Williams' "Hey good lookin' whatcha got cookin'?" His musical repertoire was impressive.

Louis never spoke unkindly about anyone or anything. He was perpetually sunny but if you were down, he shared your mood. He saw me. He understood me. He listened to me. I adored him.

We met my first year in boarding school – and when he fell in love with me, he was a year ahead and a virgin. I was not interested in having a relationship with any boy at school – the campus was too small; everyone knew everyone's business. But Louis was completely besotted with me and hard to keep at arm's length. At times it was annoying and others times, completely adorable — and it made me fall in love. But I kept pushing him away – and he never stopped coming at me in his sweet way – kind, gentle, and loving. I would get to the point where his love and constant attention were suffocating, but he never did abandon me. As I got older, I realized our connection was too intense for a couple of teenagers to handle. And I had the added deep-down feeling I was unlovable; how could this boy be so in love with me? I pushed him away because I felt I was undeserving. At those times, it annoyed me he thought I was everything.

Eventually I couldn't imagine living my life without Louis being in it. He was Jewish, and I was not, which didn't please his father, (my parents could care less) but that wasn't going to change anything. I had never met his father but he would tell me his dad was not pleased with this "shiksa," a derogatory term for a non-Jewish woman. Despite that, Louis would do anything for me. But I wished he wouldn't suffocate me. His love was too intense at times.

We continued to bond closely and became inseparable.

That first year of freedom at boarding school was a turning point. I abused the freedom without responsibility. The wide-open space on which I found myself allowed full expression for my misguided behaviors. Louis was a stabilizing factor but we were both experimenting with drugs – it was the 1970s – and a common practice among teens. I was 16, he was 17.

A friend brought a fresh batch of "window pane" LSD from NYC one weekend. A group of us agreed to trip out together. I felt more like having my own experience so I made an agreement with Louis and the others. I'd go into the woods, walk the trails, commune with nature. I'd meet them in an hour or two. It was January, it was cold and there was a deep layer of snow on the ground.

We dropped the acid and slowly scattered. The sun was out, the sky a deep cerulean blue and it was ice cold. I headed for my favorite tree in an open field on the edge of the Berkshire woods. It was a huge bare tree, full leaf in summer, but now completely barren. It was a still a magnificent silhouette of gray branches forming a perfect corona against the snow on the mountains. It was a virgin snow and no tracks, save those of small animals, could be seen anywhere on the ground.

As I walked to the tree, time warped and I lost my thought – where was I going again? It felt like an engine had been started within me and was increasing in speed and energy. Oh yeah, the tree, and I started walking again. I blanked out until I heard the Berkshire mountains begin to whisper messages to me. I could not quite hear. I was startled, and stopped – did I hear it right? What were they saying? My thoughts were ping ponging on their own and colors looked more vibrant. Everything had a vibrating halo around it in neon colors. The mountains were continuing to talk in a language I didn't understand. I couldn't decide what to focus on, and then I could not focus.

My thoughts backed up and fell upon each other in a confusing pile. I tried to sort out what I was trying to do. I was at the tree. Yes, the tree. A gust of wind blew and the branches rattled. I looked down at my feet. I saw my footprints in the snow and began walking. Time warped again, wrapped itself in a knot, and I forgot where I was. I was meandering in my mind, unaware of my body. Feeling on the edge of bliss and the screaming edge of a cliff at the same time. I had only one clear thought.

I'm meeting Louis.

Louis will be meeting me.
Louis.

I was moving again but where? In my body or my head?

Louis.

Louis.

Like a mantra it wove some kind of anchor to my building madness.

As my reality twisted, condensed into small curled-up energies, expanded out into looping tendrils, and returned to tight thoughts of nothing, the only reality I had that was true was Louis. Meeting Louis.

My thoughts jumbled and telescoped again. Small things got big, big things got small. My thoughts were out of my control and were accelerating. As I tried to ground myself, the bliss disappeared and the screaming cliff was looming.

I looked down at the snow. I had been wandering in circles under the bare branches of the big tree and going nowhere – thousands of meandering foot prints. I was the only one there.

Seeing this alarmed me. I tried very hard to gather my thoughts and move on to find Louis — my one cohesive thought – but the mountains began to talk to me again. This time it was not a whisper but a strident message of warning and urgency that I couldn't quite understand. The mountains were turning colors and their edges were vibrating. They were upset. It was some kind of warning. I was gasping for air and felt menace approaching.

A strong gust of wind blew and the tree branches above my head rattled. I looked up. The gray scaly tree branches had morphed into snakes – gray-patterned, menacing snakes, each branch rattling its fangs at me. The fear exploded and I ran. I ran across the snow-covered open field under the blue winter sky, fear pulsing out one thought: *Louis – LOUIS! LOUIS!* All other realities receded into a dark madness of thoughts wired to an approaching threat within me.

I heard "Louis!" come out of my mouth – but it was like watching a movie and hearing someone else screaming. The person screamed louder. LOUIS! LOUIS! LOUIS!

With each scream, a huge neon sign lit up in front of me with the letters of his name, mocking me. LOUIS! LOUIS!

I fell to the ground and curled in a fetal position. The screaming continued. I wondered who was screaming.

It seemed a very long time until I heard a panting sound. It echoed and ricocheted off the snow and off me. Another sound joined it. A loud thumping sound. It was very far away.

As I tried to untwist my knotted fear and scattershot thoughts, and figure out the screaming, a presence dropped heavily to my side. Heavy breathing. I was sobbing. I was the one screaming in abject fear.

I felt arms around me, hugging me. I immediately connected with a more stable reality. The presence was familiar. It was caring and loving.

It was Louis.

He was aghast at my condition. "Jules! Are you okay!? Jules, what happened?!"

He thought I was badly injured. As soon as his arms were around me, I started to come out of the very bad LSD trip. I could barely tell him what was wrong. I couldn't speak. I couldn't breathe. Finally, in between sobs, I managed to haltingly say:

"Too . . . much . . . LSD."

He hugged and held me in the snowy field on that cold winter day under the bluest sky. Louis. Louis. He was an immediate antidote. In moments the LSD effects began to lessen. I came down from the high. I felt so desolate and sorry for the experience I'd just put myself through. His love and concern brought me slowly back to reality. Thoughts began to organize and make sense. We got up and slowly walked back to my dorm. It was like a death march. What had I done?

We met up with our friends and my bad trip brought everyone out of their own high. LSD worked strangely that way.

In the weeks to follow, I reflected on what had happened. It so scared me. I felt like I would never get back to reality again – and the fear from the snakes was real and terrifying.

Being so out of control of my thoughts was a menacing feeling overwhelming me after a fairly peaceful start.

I had no one to blame for this experience but myself. I did this to myself! Me! My parents, a frequent target for my anger (I often blamed them for my life not being what I wanted) were 871 miles away.

There was no authority figure at the school to rail against, it was so liberal. No target to pin my unhappiness on, no one to blame, fight against, find revenge for. A quote from the Buddha comes to mind:

"Anger is like drinking poison and expecting the other person to die."

I had been drinking poison.

Taking drugs to get back at my parents. Engaging in taking risks to get revenge for all the teen angst I put on my mother.

At age 16, I knew without a doubt that I only had myself to blame for the bad LSD trip. I vowed to never take drugs again – nothing – no marijuana, no uppers, no downers – all the bits that students seemed to get their hands on during that time. I was out. No more. Done.

Winter passed, then spring came. I went home for the summer before my senior year at boarding school. I was reading a lot of books on spiritual traditions and I learned about a sacred word to use for chanting that brings spiritual, emotional, and mental peace. HU. I was 17 years old. I started to chant this word every night – in my walk-in closet sitting on the floor so no one would hear me. The roller coaster of my life seemed to flatten out into a calming ride toward greater understanding.

But I had to look inside myself and find the cause of my unhappiness. I discovered that the cause was me. Not my parents, not my diabetes, not my outer life. It was simply ME. It made me begin to seek answers with more urgency.

I started to explore the deeper meanings of life – and face the life I had been given. Why was I here? Who am I? I read all the books I could find on Eastern thought, and other sacred texts. Who was I and why was I here? What happens when we die? I thought again of my little sister Nancy's death, and how that affected my family. It was like a bomb going off and my mother completely shut down, emotionally wrecked. Her rigidity became more rigid, she became more controlling, as she tried to navigate the loss of a child. How I wish she could have found the comfort and peace she so sorely needed to heal from that loss. She hunkered down so low that she was not there emotionally. As a child I didn't understand this. As an adult, I weep for her. She had to walk her own path to understanding. But I wish she had the emotional support she so sorely needed, from other women, from society, from anyone.

It didn't bother Louis in the least that I no longer participated in smoking joints or refused to get high. Our connection was very deep. My decision affected him too. He was less apt to hang out doing nothing but getting high. We had private jokes that stemmed from experiences we had hiking or driving cross country when just one word would reduce us to a knowing smirk or silly laughing. It was like having your own language. We were building memories that would be cemented in each of us forever. Drugs were not a part of that nor would they ever be.

That summer before my Senior year he came and stayed with me at my parent's home for a few weeks. Separate bedrooms of course – but we found a spot behind the couch in the family room. My older sister found us there because she was letting her boyfriend out the side door after sneaking him into her bedroom in the basement.

Louis shared my interest in spiritual topics and we began to have deep conversations about life, love, death, God, and what happens after you die.

I had just read a real-life story about a woman, quite advanced in age, who made a deal with her husband on his deathbed that he would give her a sign of an afterlife once he passed. The woman was novelist Taylor Caldwell. Her husband agreed and then died. I don't remember where I read this story but found it again on the website of one Father Duffy, an Irish Catholic priest from Donegal.

>   *Taylor Caldwell was a bestselling author back in the 1950s and 1960s. For decades, her historical romances dominated the bestseller charts. In terms of sales and excitement, she was the mid-century's equivalent of Danielle Steel.*
>   *Her devoted husband, with whom she had a long and wonderful marriage, preceded her in death. His death came after a protracted illness, but both had been preparing for it. Just minutes before his death, Taylor Caldwell clutched her husband's hand and pleaded, "If there is life on the other side, I beg you, send me a sign. Let me know you are with me."*
>   *Her husband nodded his assent.*
>   *"Promise?" she begged.*

"I promise," he said, in a very weak whisper, before he passed away.

The next morning, overcome by her grief, Taylor Caldwell stepped out into her garden, seeking solace from nature as she always did. "Oh, darling," she cried out to her husband, "If only you could send me a sign that you are with me, I could try to go on. My pain is wrenching, my grief is so strong, I fear I cannot survive otherwise."

Just then, Ms. Caldwell approached a section of her garden where the ground had always proven stubbornly infertile and had never flourished like the surrounding area. As her gaze absently swept over this section, she gasped.

In the center of this section stood a rosemary bush that had not been productive for thirty years. Just the day before, when she had walked these same grounds seeking respite from her death watch, she had commented to herself how sorry she was that the bush had never thrived. But one day later, it was inexplicably in full bloom. Staring in shock and awe at the bush, Taylor Caldwell stood motionless for a long time, absorbing its message. "Thank you," she whispered fervently, "thank you. I will be able to go on, now that I know you are with me."

She had clearly been given the sign she was seeking. She told interviewers later, "You see," she explained, "rosemary means ... remembrance."

True love never dies for it pulsates with an energy that cannot be stopped, not even by death as Taylor Caldwell describes in this lovely real-life miracle.

The story of the Rosemary bush, reminiscent of the Gospel story of the fig tree (LUKE 21:29), reminded her that the love between her and her deceased husband did not die, but lived on even after his passing from this life.

—Fr. Hugh Duffy

http://www.fatherduffy.com/think-of-the-fig-tree-and-all-the-other-trees-when-you-see-their-leaves-beginning-to-appear-you-know-that-summer-is-near-2/

When I read this story in 1976, I thought it was fantastic. A real-life miracle. Proof that we don't die. I thought of Nancy. It gave me comfort. Though I felt the invisible side of life, I needed all the proof I could get. It was so easy to forget the deep thoughts and knowingness when life got complicated or messy. That veil was an iron curtain at times, sheer chiffon at others.

Because Louis and I had so many conversations about God, life, and love this seemed a perfect deal to make with him. I had no doubt we would spend the rest of our lives together. I saw us in our 80s with white hair, having lived a full life together, making memories, and sharing love. Sitting next to a stone fireplace in our easy chairs. One of us would be waiting for the other to close the deal after a full life together when death was no longer something to fear because our life had been so good.

We never talked about marriage – I was now 19, he was 20 – but it was clear we were deeply bonded and our lives would intertwine over the coming years in ways that would be revealed as time moved. Marriage was the inevitability on a far horizon.

Louis agreed to the deal – in the happy-go-lucky way he approached everything. He was known as the kind, loyal friend to all. He would give you whatever he had and never ask for anything in return. He was selfless, easy-going, and generous. He loved to laugh and looked for any underdog he could take on as a friend. He befriended the least popular, most socially awkward kids at boarding school and made them feel like they belonged, like they had a friend who would look out for them.

His eyes sparkled with adventure when I suggested the deal. He didn't back away or make a face. He was all in.

Senior year passed, Louis graduated before I did and lived off-campus. After I graduated, I wanted to take a gap year before college. I took a job in Florida drawing portraits at Disneyworld. Louis's father had a condo in Miami so he'd come visit me every month, the entire year. Before long, the year was up and we were making plans for what was next. All my plans included Louis, of course and his included me.

I had one more month at the job so Louis came for a visit before I left Florida. It began as an unusually tense visit. He seemed more determined than ever to just inhale me – and devote his every move to my happiness. I was greatly annoyed. Pissed. I needed my space. These kinds of roller coaster days wore me out – and it was as if I had no control over my reactions of wanting to just push him away. It just made him try harder.

After a few days, we got into a huge argument. It was always me who was upset, he would not do anything deliberately to jeopardize our relationship. I had enough of him that visit. It was another instance of suffocation by Louis – he was just too attached. I was not ready for such intensity. It took me years to see that I felt undeserving of such love and loyalty from him. I was unlovable. As a result, I pushed him away constantly. His need for love kept him coming back. What a pair we were!

Louis told me the song that reminded him of me the most was *Rhiannon* by Fleetwood Mac. Sadly, the lyrics show how difficult I must have been at times. But he never left me. He kept as close as I would let him.

Rhiannon rings like a bell through the night
And wouldn't you love to love her?
Takes to the sky like a bird in flight
And who will be her lover?
All your life you've never seen
Woman taken by the wind
Would you stay if she promised you heaven?
Will you ever win?
She is like a cat in the dark
And then she is to darkness
She rules her life like a fine skylark
And when the sky is starless
All your life you've never seen
Woman taken by the wind
Would you stay if she promised you heaven?
Will you ever win?
Will you ever win?

(Lyrics by Stevie Nicks)

After our big argument, he said softly he would leave on an earlier flight and give me my space. I'm sure the *Rhiannon* lyrics rang in his ears: "Will I ever win?" I had a completely surprising reaction to this news.

For an unknown reason, I did a complete turnabout and broke into tears. I was almost hysterical. Instead of the relief I usually felt at his leaving, I pleaded for him not to go. I felt such desperation. It was as if a dark grief welled up deep inside of me through my heart and out my mouth – crying and begging for him to stay. I was not a drama queen and showing this intensity of emotion was not like me. After I calmed down, he sweetly agreed not to leave but stayed the extra four days that had been planned.

Those four days were like no other time we had ever spent together. There was no tension, only deeply felt love. Love I had been so afraid of — it was so intense and full – the connection so deep, it felt so precious and magical. I finally accepted this love he had for me and allowed him to express it fully without pushing him away. I took all my armor off and stopped protecting myself. I felt worthy of his love and returned it to him from my heart.

At that time, I lived on the Gulf Coast and remember us going to the beach each day and floating in the turquoise water just hugging each other, feeling the sun and water. There was such a sense of peace in his arms.

We had our future plans mapped out. I would finish up my job in Florida. I had been accepted at art school in San Francisco. Louis would come to my parent's house in August and drive me out to my new life in the West. He was still casting about for what to do with his life. His father took him on a tour of Europe earlier that spring, hoping to interest him in some direction. He decided on culinary school. Mostly likely wherever I was. But the plan now was he'd come get me in August and drive me to California.

After those four days he flew back home to the East Coast. It was such a sunny Florida day and we both felt so happy. We got in my VW hatchback with the rusted-out floor that got my feet wet when it rained. I pulled up to the curb at the airport for departures and we both got out of the car, kissed and hugged and said sweet things.

I got back in the VW and waited for him to disappear inside the terminal. He stopped at the double doors, turned back around holding his bag with one hand, and waved at me with the other. His long dark hair was wild and curly and he had on his aviator sunglasses. I waved back and didn't drive away until the double doors slid closed behind him and he was gone. It was the last time I would ever see him.

REFLECTIONS

When our view of the world is shattered, the broken shards of life are scattered at our feet. As excruciating as it can be, we find that the pieces fit better than they ever did before. Shattering experiences cause deep reflection. For me as a young person it awakened a deep desire to understand who I was and why I was here on earth in this body.

Through the crucible of hard experiences and pain, our bodies are a stand-in for the anger and unhappiness we might experience as a young person. We blame everything and everyone around us for our unhappiness.

Juvenile diabetes was a chance to learn how to care for my body, since I was so bent on using it as a receptacle of unhappiness, instead of seeing my body as the chariot for my Soul.

Illnesses ask us to look closely at self-compassion and self-care, especially if we have brought on the woes through poor lifestyle choices.

There is always a second, third, and fourth chance. The younger you are the more chances you get. As you age, your body is less willing to keep going and demands better care. Some listen to this call and some do not. If you are reading this book, I would imagine you are listening to this call. Not that I have any answers, but perhaps my story holds some value for you.

The first limiting belief to jettison from your thoughts is that you are too old, and it's too late for you. The pathway to health is there, waiting for you, and it will be totally unique to your circumstances, life path, state of your body, and desire to get healthy.

The point is that it is possible. You can regain your health beyond what you are experiencing today.

TO JOURNAL

- What second chances have you been given?
- What shattering experiences have taught you the most? What were those lessons?
- How can you use what you learned to pursue a healthier future in body, mind, and spirit?
- What self-limiting beliefs no longer are serving you?

FIVE

DON'T GIVE ME A SIGN

Louis adored my family – which was a surprise to me, because I'd had so much to overcome. He came from a situation where wealth was the conduit for the love he was given. But what he needed, as all children do, is to know they are loved through action, words, and deeds. Not gifts, privilege, trips, and money.

His parents had divorced when he was a kid, and his wealthy father did his best, but Louis didn't get the love he needed. Meeting my family, he was immediately invested emotionally and would buy expensive cases of beer for my dad. He had a leather lead made for my sister, stamped with her horse's name on it. He would buy my little brothers matchbox race cars they collected. He would bring my mother gifts for the kitchen, knowing she cooked a lot – like a fancy gadget or a beautiful trivet. He was accepted and treated like the precious person he was to me.

My own parents married within six months of meeting. My mother was 20 and my dad was 25.

She was a cheerleader in high school, played musical instruments, wore the latest fashions and was a dark brunette.

Some of our family DNA shows Native American blood – maybe seen in my mother's high cheekbones and dark eyes. She had full lips, beautiful skin, an athletic build and an easy laugh. In early pictures of them together, her eyes fairly sparkle with joy. It's not hard to see why my dad fell in love with her.

My dad was handsome, athletic, driven, and a born entrepreneur. He was intelligent and could talk to anyone. He loved people no matter their background or social status. He wanted to know you. He loved jazz, was a championship golfer, a horseman, basketball team captain in university, and a true sports fan. He could figure out a movie's ending in the opening scenes and loved to play jokes on his daughters. He encouraged each of us to pursue a career we wanted — no matter what it was – and supported us. The boys too – they were given names my dad felt sounded great with "All American" after them. He knew my mother's limitations in going deep into conversations and feelings so he said to me when I was 18, "If you want to talk about sex, religion, or politics, talk to me, not your mother."

It was good advice.

My mother had a childhood friend, Nancy, whose family lived in a huge house that sat in the woods high above Lake Michigan. Made of stone and wood, it was beyond the dunes, surrounded by tall white birch trees, vertical stripes in the darkness of the heavy foliage in summer, disappearing against the snow in winter. Nancy's older brother, Roger (my dad), would marry my mother many years later. He was in boarding school all those years so she didn't meet him until she was in college and both were home for the summer.

My future Aunt Nancy was gentle and soft spoken — a Swedish beauty. Her father (my grandfather) and his brother had parents who came from Sweden and settled in Minnesota like many Swedish immigrants. Maybe it was the familiar cold climate.

Nancy's house was grand and full of antiques, paintings, and precious objects d'art. Despite spending a lot of time at Nancy's, my mother never felt comfortable there – it was like a museum she said. Nothing could be touched – it had an overly formal atmosphere. There were rooms on three floors and Nancy always pointed out her brother's room.

"But we can't go in there – he's away at boarding school," she said. She never saw this brother. He was like a ghost. My mom was 12. Nancy's mother was a strong independent woman and my mother never felt comfortable around her. Little did she know that this mother of her best friend would be in her future and never leave.

My mother and Nancy remained close as they graduated high school and went off to college. My mother came home from college for the summer to be with her friends, including Nancy. My mom was dating a young man from their crowd, Dan, who was friends with the never-seen brother of Nancy, Roger, who was in graduate school in Boulder. Roger was home for the summer and Dan stupidly asked him to watch over his girl – my mom - for the summer while he was away. My dad obliged and during that time they fell madly in love. Within six months, my mom and dad got married — on Christmas Eve, 1954.

Ten months later my older sister was born; 20 months later, I was born. The third daughter was Nancy named after my mom's best friend from childhood and now her sister-in-law. By the time my mother was 26 she had four children, all girls.

In the 1950s if you were not married by age 21 – despite having aspirations for an education – it was not looked upon kindly. Something must be wrong with a woman who is not married by then. And though I know my mother loved my dad and he adored her (to the very end) she gave up her dreams of a career and getting her degree to marry him. Suddenly within five years she was a housewife with four children, stuck at home caring for us.

Many women from that era had this difficult scenario to live through and put aside dreams and desires for a full life outside of marriage and children and instead became housewives and mothers. I believe this contributed to my mother's anger and inability to process feelings. She felt caged, stuck and frustrated – though my father provided well, loved her adoringly, was supportive and caring – but to be thwarted in what you truly want your life to be was hard for her, I am sure.

Then on top of that to lose a child to cancer. My compassion and respect for my mother has grown so much as I have stepped back to look at the cards she was dealt in this life.

My father grew up in a privileged environment, his father was Swedish, his mother traced lineage back to the Mayflower. We called our grandparents Dodi and Bamps. My dad was born a few years after his older brother died at age two from an infection. Dodi was told she could not have any more children. But then here came my dad. My grandmother was born in 1904 and women of her era didn't talk about pregnancies. It was shrouded in mystery or at least was a very private experience. My father always wondered if he was actually secretly adopted. This made his sister Nancy, scoff later in life because she *had* been adopted.

Bamps was a successful businessman who made his fortune during the World War II. Too old to be drafted, so like many men at that time, he engaged in the emerging industries. He had accounts with the steel mills around Gary, Indiana. He was a very handsome man who loved to dress formally – and had a kind, loving, heart. He was larger than life and in girth. He had a brother, Daddy Chuck, who was his physical opposite. Small, wiry, and thin. But he looked out for his brother, Chuck. Daddy Chuck was twice widowed as a middle-aged man. With his first wife he had Phyllis, my aunt. After Phyllis's mom died, Daddy Chuck remarried. He and his second wife had Nancy, my Aunt and my mom's best friend. When his second wife died, he was left to raise two young girls under the age of 10. Dodi and Bamps stepped in and invited Daddy Chuck to live with them along with his daughters. Daddy Chuck and Bamps were in business together so it was a perfect solution. And thus, the name "Daddy Chuck." My grandparents eventually adopted the girls and raised them as their own. My dad gained two sisters just like that. He was so thrilled he bought Phyllis a bike with his allowance.

Nancy was younger and eventually my father was sent away to boarding school for high school. So, he was absent when his sister's friend, my mom, was around.

Once my parents met, fell in love and married, Bamps was so kind to his son's new wife. He loved my mother. But the mother-in-law relationship had tensions. The overly formal mother of her friend Nancy was now in her life permanently. Sparks flew over the decades – but as women did back then, the sparks were under the radar – it was all subtext – but you could cut the tension with a knife. Bamps, on the other hand, represented a safe harbor, love and acceptance. I think my mother needed that in her life, to know she was cherished and would be watched out for, even though my dad filled that bill as well.

My job in Florida ended and I returned to my parent's house in Indiana to await Louis who would drive me out West to art college. It was June 1976, a warm summer evening, and I had just returned from dinner with a friend. My parents had also just arrived home from dinner out with the small boys. Then the phone rang. My mother answered and said, "It's for you – I think it's Louis." The operator would always say long distance for the person being called. If you weren't there, the caller would not be charged for the call.

I ran downstairs to the basement phone for privacy.

"Hello? Louis?"

"Jules… it's Cheryl."

Something was wrong. Cheryl was my best friend from boarding school who grew up in New York City and one of the close circle of friends Louis and I were part of.

"What's wrong, Cheryl? Is everything all right?"

"Jules, are you sitting down?"

"No, should I?"

"Yes."

Then she just blurted it:

"Louis is dead."

In that moment I hated Cheryl so much I couldn't bear it. What was wrong with her! I hated her so much for saying it! My anger rose in a wave of shock and screaming like I was vomiting out my entire being.

I looked at the phone receiver in disbelief, anger, and disgust and threw it on the ground. I screeched a primal call of pain: "NOOOOOOOOOOOOO!!!!"

In a strange quietness, I felt part of me step outside my screaming self, look back at me and say:

"But you knew this was going to happen. "

On the deepest level it felt true. It anchored me more to the moment as right then my father bounded down the stairs and took the phone. Cheryl was crying and told my dad what she told me. I stopped screaming but was crying so hard I couldn't hear. My father put the phone down, grabbed me and hugged me hard and long.

He whispered in my ear, "Don't ask why, honey."

I knew Cheryl must still be on the phone. I picked it back up and simply asked:

"How?"

"He was hit on the Massachusetts turnpike. He was hitch-hiking home in the rain. In the dark. His car broke down. It was a hit-and-run."

Oh god, not Louis. Not Louis. Not Louis.

"The funeral is this weekend, Jules."

Between sobs, I said, "I'm coming. "

I had never even met his father – only his mother one time in Florida. I doubted she would remember me. She was so removed from Louis's life.

As the shock of his death hung on me, all I could think of that night was we had made a deal. It was only six months ago. That deal? Whoever went first would give the other a sign there was an afterlife.

I didn't want to know if there was an afterlife – I didn't care if there was an afterlife. I only cared about one thing. WHY?! I wanted to know why he had to die. WHY?! Even though my father had advised not to ask – that's all I did ask.

A close friend came over to spend the night in my room. I don't know what I was expecting but I needed someone close to me who could understand my pain and grief. My parents had loved Louis and knew what he meant to me, but the feelings I was showing were so intense, my mother couldn't handle it. She put my two brothers in the car and they took off as soon as I started screaming from the phone call. Years later, one of my brothers told me they didn't understand what was going on – she just fled with them. Maybe she didn't want them to see me crying hysterically.

That night I dreamed I was dragging a wooden coffin on my back, going around a small medieval village saying "Louis is dead, Louis is dead." It was a dream in dark browns and grays – stone buildings in a small village under a dark gray sky. A bell in the distance was slowly gonging. It was like a horror movie but also like a bad movie set.

I awoke the next morning in disbelief. My grief was so deep and wide it felt completely unreal. The world was a different place now. There was no Louis. How could there be no Louis?

In the 1970s, like the 1960s when Nancy died, there was no bereavement counseling. I got no real help from my parents. They were in shock too, and it was time for me to go off to San Francisco without Louis. I started college in a daze of complete desolation and grief; it took all the joy of life out of me. Settling in San Francisco, the foghorns, the sound of the public electric buses, the clanging cable cars — all bring back through sound, the terrible grief and sadness I had for years living there after losing Louis, who had been the love of my life up to that point.

REFLECTIONS

We come into this life with such a clean slate as babies – no social conditioning just eyes of wonder, and sometimes frustration at being in this small body that can't talk or walk yet. Regardless of what happens in the next 18 years, challenging childhood, self-esteem issues, weight struggles, broken love relationships, hard times … there is always the chance for more change we don't ask for.

Life can slam us to our knees and while we get our bearings, the world is dark. I learned early that life was uncertain and I had to find a way to survive anything that came along. I made choices that protected my feelings, vulnerability, and comfort zone – even though I was a risk-taker and I didn't always make the right choices.

I was engulfed in grief on a level I had not experienced before when Louis died. To avoid the pain, my body sought a self-medicating strategy – that activated the reward circuitry in my brain.

According to psychology, humans are motivated by two things:
Necessities: food, sleep, avoidance of pain
Rewards: object, event, or activity that elicits pleasure

The brain's reward system reinforces behavior associated with "rewards" and prevents behaviors associated with "punishment." The neurotransmitter Dopamine is released during rewards, and we find ways to avoid the punishment.

The painful emotions of grief and loss were punishing to say the least, and eating food, way more than I needed, often sugary sweet and poison for a Type 1 diabetic, released dopamine in my system. Food as reward to avoid painful emotions. It didn't matter that it created havoc for my blood sugar and contributed long term to many of the diabetes complications I experienced later.

Without even noticing, I put on 30 pounds my first year of college.

Emotional eating has "motivation/reward" all over it. It's an ingrained mindset needing resetting.

A painful emotion ("punishment") would motivate us to look for a "reward", i.e., FOOD. This releases dopamine in the system and temporarily stops the pain (punishment.) The brain's reward system initiates this behavior each time we have an emotional upset, reinforcing a negative relationship with food, making us unhealthy.

For some, ANY emotion is painful, even happy ones, and emotional eating can include bingeing after happy news.

Our brains are delicate organs that need proper care & feeding. Nutrient deficiencies can cause brain dysfunction. But the brain can also create new pathways thru neuroplasticity – we can change!

Feed your body essential nutrients, start moving, get blood flowing, muscles activated, and you might see how powerful your motivation is because now, you are experiencing the reward.

TO JOURNAL

- Are you an emotional eater?
- What strategies could you use to short-circuit the need for a food reward when you are upset?
- Remember how powerful your thoughts are and your use of imagination.
- Be kind to yourself and give yourself grace while you navigate this challenge.
- What supportive advice would you give a deeply loved one about how to pivot away from food rewards to something else in order to feel better?

SIX

FOR THE LOVE OF AUNTS

When Louis died my life became a dark place of sorrow. Along with his mother and father, he had an older brother, but Louis struggled with finding his place in a career. However, the older brother was a business genius. I have read about him as one of the wealthy one percent - due to the sale of a business that hit the market with a corporate buyer at just the right time in the 1990's. He is probably the only person still living who remembers Louis. I don't remember any cousin's names or aunts or uncles. I have no information there. But his brother is still living. I wrote him a letter a couple of years ago, but didn't mail it. His wealth is so extreme I doubted that he would get it, read it, or even consider its meaning.

That first weekend after I got the news was utterly devastating. Cheryl, a dear friend Louis and I shared from Stockbridge, told me where and when the funeral would be. It was to be a traditional Jewish service. My dad got some money out of his office safe to buy me a plane ticket to New York. I would stay with Cheryl. Louis would be buried in New Jersey near where his father lived.

I had never met his father. I knew he did not approve of me because I was a chiksa (non-Jewish) but that didn't bother me. Louis and I had been together for three years and I didn't see that ever ending. I was his first love – literally – and he wrote me letters expressing sentiments about that. I wrote letters back. We went on road trips and took lots of pictures with instamatics. Louis went to Europe with his dad the spring before he died and they had the best time. He sent postcards and told me what a great time he was having. His father had always been disapproving of Louis in general – as the older brother was such a go-getter. Louis was just like so many kids during that time – trying to figure it out. The trip to Europe was a way for Louis to bond with his father, who thought Louis was struggling to find his way in life.

I was packing for the funeral when the phone rang. It was Louis's father.

In his deep, gravelly voice, he said,

"Julia, this is Louis's father. The funeral is in two days. I want to pay your ticket. You will stay with me. I will take care of everything. I won't take no for an answer."

I said, "Thank you, Mr. R. I was planning to come. My friend Cheryl was going to pick me up. My dad already bought me a ticket."

Mr. R said, "Tell your friend I am going to take care of everything. Let me speak to your father."

Louis's father and my dad spoke at length. Mr. R told him how much it meant that my parents treated Louis like family. Louis had talked about my dad all the time, how great he was, how kind.

So it was decided. Louis's father would pick me up at the airport and take care of everything. I had no idea what to expect. I was in a daze on the plane . . . how could this be — Louis is dead? He was so full of life and I needed to be with my friends who all knew and loved Louis. We needed to grieve together.

I arrived at the airport and there was no one to pick me up. Then I saw a man holding a sign with my name on it. I headed over to him and he asked, "Are you Julia? I'm 'sposed to take you to Fort Lee to Mr. R's building." I said okay and we got into the town car and drove off.

The New York skyline was visible from the highway. It looked cold, grey, and overwhelming despite the summer heat. After 45 minutes, we arrived at a luxury high-rise building overlooking the Hudson River. The driver got out, dropped my bags on the pavement, said thank you and drove off. I went into the lobby.

"Can I help you?" a doorman asked.
"I'm here for Mr. R. He's expecting me."
"Oh, he just left."
"What?"
"He just left."
"To go where?"
"I don't know."
The desk phone rang.
"Excuse me," said the doorman. He held the phone in one hand, looked up and said, "Are you Julia?"
I said, yes, and he jabbed the receiver toward me.
"It's for you."

"Hello?"
"Is this Julia?"
"Yes."

"This is Louis's aunt. Max had to leave. I'm so sorry. Can you get a taxi to meet us at a hotel in Orange, New Jersey? I'll give you the address. "

I had just flown for hours, was exhausted and bereft, and this was no comfort.

"Can I go upstairs to the apartment just to use the powder room?" I asked the aunt.

"No, don't go upstairs, please. I'll explain later. Just get a taxi."

Her voice was kind and soothing so I asked the doorman to call me a taxi.

But I did go upstairs. I don't remember how – maybe the doorman let me in. I was in the apartment for only a brief moment.

I entered the living room and my letters to Louis and our pictures were all over the low glass coffee table. A woman in her early 40's was sitting on the couch. She had red eyes and spoke with a heavy Eastern European accent. She seemed very upset but also vulnerable. We didn't converse much; I just kind of came in and left after using the bathroom. I was shocked to see my letters to Louis and our photos on the table but said nothing.

Downstairs, the taxi was waiting.

We were driving to the hotel in Orange and the taxi driver asked me cheerfully, "So are you here on vacation?"

In my 19-year-old heart I thought, *How do I begin to tell him what is going on in this unfolding drama?*

"No," I said and fell silent.

We got to the hotel. As I stepped out of the taxi, the glass double doors opened up and a line of five women my mother's age with arms linked were marching toward me. When they got close, their arms unlinked and were outstretched. I was enveloped in the love and care of Louis's Jewish aunts who welcomed me like a long-lost daughter. I began to cry, and they ushered me to a car. One held my hand and it was clear they all felt my pain and grief. Louis's father must have told them all about us.

We arrived at one of his aunt's homes. It was palatial. All I wanted to do was sleep. I was given a quiet and beautifully appointed guest room after meeting some of Louis's cousins. They all said how special Louis was and how sorry they were about his death. They all knew what we meant to each other. The letters and pictures had shown the true nature of our love for each other and it moved his family to know that Louis had someone in his life like me. His father especially.

One of the aunts said to me at the house, "Louis's father, Max, is so strong. He is the rock in this family. He's so strong. We all depend on him." The other aunts all nodded in agreement, "He is, he is." "He's so strong." I didn't know how it would go, but all I wanted was to cry on his shoulder. Louis's father. He would understand better than anyone else this deep loss.

The aunt whose home it was sat up with me for a long time that night before I went to bed and listened to my stories about Louis and how much I loved him. How much grief and pain I was in now that he was gone. She was like an angel and I will always remember her caring deeply about how I felt. She treated me like a valued daughter.

I still had not met his father. The aunt explained to me that Max had a girlfriend who was younger and not mentally strong. She had gone with him to identify Louis's body in Massachusetts and freaked out. There was a terrible scene when they came back to the New Jersey apartment. Max had to leave. The aunt ended with, "The girl friend is crazy."

Finally, I went to sleep in the lovely guest room with hardwood floors and matching drapes and bedspread. The funeral was going to be the next day. In the morning, still asleep, I felt myself hovering above my body sleeping on the bed – a new sensation – and I could "see" Louis's dark-haired cousin walking down the hall, then gently knocking on my door, which woke me. She opened the door and said, "Good morning." I opened my eyes and there she was in the flesh.

REFLECTIONS

There is no such thing as old age, just age.

No one needs to just give up and give in.

We know what goes around comes around because our bodies wear it.

We have an invisible shield that surrounds us — an aura — made up of our energy and vibrations created by our thoughts, feelings, and desires. That aura attracts similar energies — in people and situations.

Whether expectations in life are mindful and conscious or unconscious, the Universe will bring it. That's our secret SUPERPOWER.

The aura can be made strong & healthy so that negativity bounces right off — or it can be so weak that toxic people affect us and live rent-free in our heads.

Making an agreement with yourself is a sacred pact – an agreement to get fit, get healthy, take better care of your body.

How many times did I violate the health of my body through mindless actions? Every time we break a sacred pact with ourselves, we open a hole in our aura for more of what we are transforming OUT OF to get BACK IN.

Our auras are the result of MINDSET work. Or lack of it.

Love, gratitude, morning meditations, and daydreaming positive visions can strengthen our aura, creating a path for a stronger mindset.

Pair that with day-in, day-out repetitive positive actions, such as lifting weights, cardio, and eating nutrient dense food and YOU WILL COMPLETELY TRANSFORM — in ways way beyond your physical temple of a body.

Jump on that energy & ride it into your transformation. Our fitness journeys are a good way to test out these ideas.

Be patient, your body needs time to transform. Keep the SACRED PACT with yourself to get healthy, strong and vibrant.

Your SUPERPOWER awaits conscious activation. BANG BANG!!

Because actually we are AGELESS.

And just when you think you cannot go another step, find the next open door, the Universe, God, whatever you call the Divine, will send you the equivalent of five loving Aunts who will embrace you to their very hearts, and carry you as far as they need to.

When the student is ready, the teacher appears.

TO JOURNAL

- When has the right person showed up in your life to help you take the next step?
- Write down a composite description of the "shero," mentor, coach or being with whom you can trust, learn from, and help you reach your goals.
- What qualities do they have?
- What do you want them to teach you?

SEVEN

MY SON, MY SON!

The funeral home was some miles away. I needed to see my friends. Cheryl knew that Louis's father had picked me up so I didn't get to spend the night and grieve with her. I got to the funeral home early with the aunts. Finally, I saw Cheryl and all our friends. We held on tight, hugging and crying. I glanced up at the opening to the room the service was in. Louis's name was above the door to the inner sanctuary – it was real and unreal at the same time.

As we stood together, a handsome, spry man with a full head of white hair, deeply lined crevices on his face, and intense eyes under bushy brows, entered the funeral home and came straight for me.

Louis's father, Max.

"Julia?"
"Yes?"
"Walk with me."
No preamble, no greeting. Just "walk with me."
He took my arm and we went outside. It was a modest New Jersey neighborhood. We headed down the block and

I started to cry – who else but his father could understand and share my grief? To my surprise he said, "No! Let me!"

As we put distance between us and the funeral home, he began to wail and keen, saying over and over: "My son! My son!" He was beside himself. I remained silent, holding back tears in the face of the raw grief of a man who has lost his 20-year-old son in a hit-and-run.

We kept walking for blocks. He eventually calmed down. Wiping tears and blowing his nose with a handkerchief, he told me how grateful he was that I made his son a man – a way of saying he knew I was Louis's first love.

He said, "I found your letters and pictures and could see how important you were to each other. Thank you for loving my son."

Though I never worried about his father's disapproval of me, to have this recognized by him was a gift.

He continued, "You'll sit with me during the service in the front row. I want you to ride with me to the cemetery. You'll be in the car with me. Louis's mother is very upset, you won't want to be around her. "

I remembered the time I had met her in Florida with her second husband. She had dyed, bright red hair, red fingernails, and red lipstick. The second husband was wearing a Hawaiian shirt, yellow slacks, and white, patent-leather loafers. We had lunch with them and she offered me some noodle kugel – a delicious Jewish dish full of butter and sugar. I declined.

"Why?" she asked.

"I'm diabetic."

Her husband piped up, suddenly interested in me, "Do you take shots in the butt?"

Yes, I would avoid her.

We got back to the funeral home and Max asked me if I would read the eulogy at the service for Louis. I said I would. But I thought a moment and asked, "Can I just say something in my own words – instead of reading something?"
He said, "Of course."

We walked back to the funeral home and went into the room where Louis's closed casket was. The room looked like a large terrarium – glassed in on all sides with plants and greenery around the coffin, like in a forest. Flowers were in the foyer but not here.

The service started as I sat in the front row with Max. A rabbi trained in music, a cantor, sang the most beautiful song in Hebrew. It lasted for about 10 minutes. I was then invited to get up and speak.

I thought of all our friends sitting there and how we knew Louis and his pure heart and giving, generous nature. I knew his father had labeled him a messed-up kid and thought he was not going to make anything of himself like his brother had. The brother did not attend the funeral because he was in the Bahamas.

I wanted the cousins, aunts and uncles to know the true nature of Louis as a giving heart and how much we loved him. As I spoke his father wept and shook his head up and down in agreement at my words. I found words to say that I had not thought to say beforehand.

I remember saying:

"Louis had the biggest heart of anyone I knew. He was kind, generous and accepted everyone no matter what. He would give you all he had if you needed it. He loved nature, so this setting is very appropriate for Louis. But the body that lies here is not Louis. Louis was soul. He won't just live on in our memories, but he is an eternal being and so he lives on, not just in our hearts but as a living Soul."

I don't know where I got the words. But I believed every word I said as it came out of my mouth. It was as if a part of me knew things I didn't consciously understand. I felt strong and open and wanted to share the reality of this young man whose life had been taken by a hit-and-run driver. I loved Louis so much.

I felt joy as I spoke and later said to Cheryl, "I could feel Louis pinching my butt!" We both laughed. I really felt his joyous, playful presence. But the dark veil of grief would descend again and stay for decades to come.

We drove to the cemetery and the service was over. I left with my friends to go over to another aunt's house to sit shiva – the mirrors were covered in the house in the Jewish tradition.

I flew home a day later and felt the emptiness of the future without him. No one talked about him at home. Though my parents had loved him, they probably didn't want to upset me. But it was like he never existed.

A week later, his older brother called me. He must have felt the guilt settle on his shoulders for not attending his brother's funeral. He asked me: "What did Louis think of me?"

Frankly, Louis never talked about his brother. I had the urge to tell him what I thought of him – for not coming to the service – but I knew it might be something he would carry for the rest of his life, so I said, "He loved you very much, respected you, and talked about you a lot."

I thought again about the deal Louis and I made. It no longer seemed to matter – if there was an afterlife or not. He was gone, that's all I knew.

It was within that year I knew I had a choice to make. I was angry at God for taking Louis away from me. My seeking and searching for life's answers had simply become too large to handle and I fell back on blaming God for my pain and grief. But in that year, as I had after the bad LSD trip at age 16, I faced myself and knew I had to choose. Would I be a victim of this loss and blame God forever and be bitter? Or would I move forward and trust there were answers in life that I didn't have yet — answers that would eventually give me peace.

I chose to move forward and trust life. Though I still had a fear of living that was to come out again later, for now, I would take charge of my happiness and try to find the good that was waiting for me.

Within months of that decision, almost a year after he died, I had a very lucid dream with Louis. I woke up the next morning and it was as if I had spent an entire day on the beach with him like we did in Florida. I was so full of love and contentment waking up from being with him in the dream. My heart was so full. He had met me on a steep sloping mountain and showed me the cabin he lived in. He was joyous and silly, and kept saying over and over: "Life is

Great! Life is Great!" I tried to interject, "But you died ..."
and he would simply ignore that and say again, "Life is Great!"

That was my sign from Louis, that there was an afterlife.
He made good on our deal.

The pain of losing him has never really abated on a deep
level. I still think of him often and mourn the life he did not
get to live. The only person I knew who would understand the
depth of this loss was his father. We stayed in touch and when
I lived in New York City later, he would take me to dinner.

As time passed, and I moved West, I would write him and
he'd write back. He sent pictures of his two granddaughters
by his other son. And photos of his current girlfriend. I just
wanted him to know that someone on this earth still deeply
loved his son and thought about him almost every day. It was
like Louis was just "with me" inside and never left. Even my
dear husband Paul understood this and the picture of Louis
I carried in my wallet. They would have been great friends.

There were times I called his father just to say "Hi." I had
his office number and his assistant would answer. As soon as
I said my name, she would get Max on the phone. He would
not even say hello, he'd be sobbing and wailing "My son!
My son!" just as he did outside the funeral home so many
decades earlier. The assistant would take back the phone and
say kindly, "I'm sorry, Max just can't talk right now."

I couldn't bear to upset him like that anymore so I stopped
calling and sent my love and well wishes invisibly and in letters. A couple of years ago I got a nudge to call the number I
had for him and a woman answered. I asked if I could speak
to Mr. R. She said, "I'm very sorry, but Mr. R has been in a

nursing home now for several years." He must have been in his 90's by then.

I hung up and started watching obituaries for his name to come up. And one day it did. I was deeply touched to see the small paragraph say he had now joined his beloved son, Louis, who died in 1976. Thank God someone acknowledged and remembered this special Soul, my Louis.

REFLECTIONS

Life can change in a moment. We go along as if nothing will ever be exciting again in a bored state of acceptance. Or we go along with grief trailing us wherever we go when we are blindsided with something that only happens to other people. These heavy emotional tolls exact payment. It's a roller-coaster ride of emotional upheaval which is excellent practice for managing our thoughts, feelings, and desires. Pain teaches us to find another way once we get tired of the effects coming our way. We can't control the death of a loved one from a hit-and-run, of course we can't. But we can control how we react to it. Initially the grief and pain are overwhelming, but how does time manage to soothe the wound? We think about it less; the pain of loss subsides, as life moves, and the thing we think about is the love that was shared and is left with us by this wonderful Soul.

It may not be something that can be consciously worked on, but it's the path by which I learned to redirect thoughts from dark to light. My question of WHY became a feeling of gratitude for what I shared with Louis while he was alive. What he taught me about myself, how he treated me.

"It's amazing, Molly. The love inside, you take it with you."
— Sam in the film *Ghost,* directed by Jerry Zucker (1990).

There is always a new lesson to be learned, ready to roll down the pipeline of our life. As the grief was overtaken by love memories of Louis, the childhood diabetes caught up with me and began to ravage my body.

TO JOURNAL

- Describe one or two significant events in your life that have transformed you into who you are today.
- When do you trust yourself most?
- When do you find it harder to have faith in your ability to realize your goals?
- Complete this sentence and keep writing: "I need to accept that _____."
- Write a letter to someone you've lost, whether they've died or simply drifted away from your life. What do you have left to tell them?

EIGHT

BLINDNESS COMES IN MANY FORMS

I n the late 1970's and early 1980's, San Francisco was a dark time of grief, and also a time that diabetes complications began to appear in my body. In my apartment, I had Japanese shoji screens in my bedroom to let light in, but provide privacy from close neighbors whose windows faced mine. I woke up one morning and the white grid squares of the shoji screen had a huge black spot in the center which moved when I moved my eyes. My overall vision was blocked by a dark spot – I could only see in my peripheral vision, with no central vision.

I was terrified that I had awakened blind.

Recently, my diabetic doctor told me my kidneys were starting to fail and in the next 10 years would have to face being on dialysis. These were the realities of living with diabetes from childhood. I was a "brittle" case, or labile; my blood sugars were hard to control no matter what I did or how well I took care of myself. My blood sugars would bounce all over the place. The high glucose in my blood wore away the vascular lining and caused small blood vessels to leak – first the eyes, then the kidneys where they are smallest.

I called my father, hysterical. He calmed me down and said to find an eye doctor right away, which I did.

The black spot in my eye cleared by the afternoon. I got to the eye doctor, who knew I was diabetic. He labeled it an "ocular migraine." Nothing to worry about. I'll never forget that bogus diagnosis. "Ocular Migraine."

It happened again and again, so I went to a highly regarded eye specialist. His diagnosis: I had proliferative diabetic retinopathy in both eyes. It would require laser surgery to cauterize the leaking blood vessels which were a diabetic complication. I would go blind if they did not start immediately. It meant getting small laser burns in both eyes – I had about 3,000 burns in each eye. I was 24 years old.

The procedure was done in the doctor's office, but was grueling. They gave me a sedative and then the doctor's long-time nurse, Betty, would come and inject a local anesthetic into the hollow below my eye socket. As I lay on the table, she would wiggle her fingers above my head and slightly to the back so I would have to look up and back – and not see the needle coming. Then she would deftly push the needle into the hollow below my eye and above my cheekbone as I took deep halting breaths. The doctor would then shoot lasers through my retina and cauterize the tiny blood vessels to stop the bleeding. Afterwards my eyes would be sore and very sensitive to light. The bright California sun was agonizing. I could barely see. My aunt Nancy lived in Carmel and I took the bus to be with her. She took care of me until I got better.

My father realized what a hard time I was having in San Francisco so he flew out to see me, and his sister Nancy. At one point he took my shoulders and looked me in the eye. With the kind of energy only a dad can muster, he said, "Honey, you can't go before me. Please promise me that."

He knew the situation was dire with my diabetes and I had a long road ahead. He had already lost one daughter, and could not bear to lose another. My mother felt the same but was unable to express it. But I knew she was terrified of the same thing happening.

Around that time, I was also investigating all kinds of healing modalities that might make my health better. A book had come out called *Healing Ourselves: A Book to Serve as a Companion in Time of Illness and Health* by a Japanese doctor, Naboru Muramoto. Based on Asian medicine and his teachings, it was a popular book at the time. He was seeing patients in the basement of a local church. I made an appointment and found this small Japanese man in the musty church basement with stacked folding chairs and a rickety table.

He was chain-smoking. His English was halting. I tried to explain that I was diabetic. The first thing he did was motion to my bosom, laugh, and make hand signs signaling his approval at their size. Christ. Then he told me to stop taking my insulin and take these little black pills instead. I knew better. That was it for Dr. Muramoto.

The first glucometer came out around this time in the mid-1980's. I could now rely on real-time blood-sugar readings, not dipsticks into urine samples that were hours old and inaccurate.

The insulin pump was also a new device that diabetics could wear around their waist. It would administer insulin at the touch of a button. The device had a tube hooked up to a syringe with a subcutaneous needle in your belly at all times. I got one – anything to help manage my diabetes better.

It was the size of a medium paperback book. I had to wear a belt all the time in order to carry it with me. Once getting on a plane, the security guard insisted I take it off and out – she had never seen one before.

As a result of having an excess of insulin all the time, my body began to efficiently store food as fat. I gained so much weight and look bloated and round. My sister's wedding pictures from that time really show the suffering I was going through, trying to manage my diabetes any way I could. Finally, the pump had to go. It was not working for me. I switched to multiple shots per day.

Once my health stabilized from changing from the insulin pump to multiple insulin shots (up to 6 a day) I began to feel better. I had more energy and food was metabolizing more normally without the excess insulin in my system. I moved to New York City. I started doing exciting freelance work and found a great job. I had an endocrinology specialist, Dr. Mirsky, a doctor who later ended up saving my life. But as I walked to work every day on the streets of Manhattan, I noticed the chic, slim women around me, who looked beautiful and effortless in their slender bodies. I felt so inadequate and so unattractive. It was intimidating. I was also unhappy on a deep level and I blamed this on my being overweight.

If I could only lose the weight, I'll be happy, I thought. *I'll fit into this chic stream of young professional beauties I pass every day and feel like I belong here.* I found a book called – *The Pineapple Diet* and that lasted a week. Too much sugar from the fruit and not enough to slow down the glycemic reaction from eating the pineapples.

Then another book: *A Woman Doctor's Diet for Women.* It was basically a keto diet – an early Dr. Atkins, feminine version. I coupled that with running every night around the streets near my apartment for 30 minutes. In about three months I had released the weight I wanted to lose. But I was also experiencing terrible cramps and diarrhea from too much protein and no carbs. The worst part was after losing the weight, I was still unhappy. I thought if I lost weight, I would be happy – but I was the same unhappy person in a skinnier body.

It was here that my feelings of unworthiness and low self-esteem got real.

I went with a friend after work to a nightclub. As we ate appetizers and danced, I noticed a man watching me. He was alone and looked a bit older but was definitely handsome. He came over and asked me to dance. He was also very charming. He was tall, dark, and lanky with the body of an athlete, and his dark eyes shone like black coal. He had an easy laugh, but also had a look of being tightly wound. Like a spring ready to pop off. I was very attracted but I didn't give him my number. My friend and I were going to dinner. I told him where, then we left. Halfway through dinner, he showed up, which I thought was bold of him. We continued our conversation. One thing led to another and we began a relationship.

At this point in my life, I was attracted to the "bad boys." They were a little edgy, hyper masculine, and tough. I eventually realized it was a symptom of low self-esteem to attract men who would treat me poorly. It was the way I thought I deserved to be treated. It was so subconscious and I was so unaware of this within myself that I walked into a relationship with Sam without trepidation or caution.

At first it was such a strong physical attraction. But there were warning signs about his temper that I ignored. He also seemed to drink a lot. I was 27, he was 39. At one point I could see that his lifestyle was not meshing with mine – I was not a drinker and his life was all about nightclubs and bars. I told him I couldn't see him anymore if that was his lifestyle – because it wasn't mine. He seemed to quit drinking alcohol overnight.

The relationship continued and I felt less alone in the big city of New York as a single woman in her twenties. Mostly what we spent time doing is a blurred memory. We had little in common besides the physical attraction. I had a good job and was confident in my life so when he asked me to marry him, I wasn't sure. He brought it up – getting married. It wasn't really a proposal and I didn't immediately agree.

Note to self: if you are asked to marry someone, and you have to wonder about saying yes or no, then the answer is NO. I asked God what to do. I got a visual in my head of a green traffic light which to me meant, yes, go ahead. So, I did.

It was not a big wedding, it was just me, my parents, and my best friend, Cheryl. Oddly my mother picked the church in New York City that was in line with her denomination and I allowed this. We showed up to the old Manhattan church on a Saturday, and met with the priest. It was a dark, musty church with a sanctuary bearing the energy of untold supplications and prayers. He looked Irish. He had gray hair, was portly and was wearing a collar as priests do. He looked Catholic, but he was Presbyterian, my mother's denomination.

I was ready to just sign the papers and be done with the ceremony so I asked, "Where do you want us?"
He said, "Not so fast."

He had us sit down in his church office and proceeded to lecture us for 30 minutes on marriage and the challenges we would face living in NYC. How marriage was sacred and we should honor each other . . . he went on and on, mostly platitudes, but we listened respectfully. Finally, he said we could go to the sanctuary and indeed the ceremony took only a few minutes after the 30-minute lecture.

Ever since I was a child, I felt there was someone out there for me – waiting to meet up and share love and life together. I thought of this someone as "the one." The love of my life to be. After Louis died, I had a stronger sense of it. It was not a concrete thought, just a fleeting feeling in my heart that would sit there quietly despite my choices in men, after Louis.

This feeling lived outside my emotional attachments to men to whom I was attracted to. The slightly hard-edged "bad boys" and semi-dangerous-looking masculine types – it was an attraction that exercised itself beyond my control. When I met Sam, he had that "look." Besides being handsome, he was wound pretty tight and held himself like a football player, which is what he had been, a semi-pro. He was the opposite of Louis in every way. It had been eight years since Louis's death.

After the lecture with the priest, we moved into the sanctuary. My dad walked me down the aisle and as he handed me over to be married, I looked at Sam and this thought came into my head: *He's not "the one."*

It wasn't a shocking thought; it was a fact – and I was emotionally detached from its meaning. It was like information to be stored away – like the Universe had just whispered this in my ear and added, "Just so you know..."

After the ceremony, before we left to go to a favorite restaurant, Sam leaned over out of earshot of my parents and said, "That priest was drunk."

I protested, "No, he wasn't! He didn't act it and he didn't smell like alcohol."

What did Sam know anyway?

At the restaurant, we sat at a round table, with my mother next to Sam. I glanced at the two of them and had the oddest feeling and sensation that they looked alike. I filed that away quickly and didn't think of it again.

We married in May and a month later my youngest brother came for a visit. We lived in a Brooklyn brownstone and decided to take a walk to show him our neighborhood. We crossed streets and turned corners and passed brownstones with stoops and people sitting out in the sun. It was a sunny New York summer day.

We came upon two older men sitting outside their building. As we got closer, I saw it was the priest who had married us a month before. I rushed over to say hello and called Tom, my brother, over to meet the priest.

After an enthusiastic "Hi!" from me, I got a blank look from the priest who was in street clothes. He said hesitating. "Hello?"

"Don't you remember me?" I motioned to Sam who was standing behind me.

"No, should I?" said the priest.

"Yes, you married us a month ago at your church."

He was embarrassed now and said, "You must have been dressed differently. "

Dumbfounded, we walked away. I said to Sam, "After that long lecture and he didn't remember us?"
Sam replied, "I told you he was drunk."
What kind of message was the Universe sending me about this marriage?

REFLECTIONS

Nothing outside of ourselves is going to be the source of our happiness. A thinner body, a love relationship, a new job, house, partner … whatever. The happiness comes from deep inside and ATTRACTS exactly what is needed in your life "out here." I put the price of my happiness on a relationship and handed it to a man who did not handle it with any care at all. I deliberately but unconsciously chose a man who treated me the way I felt I deserved to be treated: worthlessly. Without respect. Trampled feelings, physical and verbal abuse. We sleepwalk through trauma doing the best we can, even though we are our own jailers with the key to get out of prison. Free once and for all. I had no idea the power I had to create a life of my dreams. I had created a life of nightmares based on my low self-esteem. Either way, the energy we project and live by will manifest in our life as outer conditions. We look around and ask "Why me? What did I do to deserve this?" Actually, a lot. And I don't mean in the way the abuser wants his victim to feel like it's her fault. I mean in the deep recesses of your being, saying I AM WORTHY OF LOVE, RESPECT and HAPPINESS. Getting it can be a long, painful journey of discovery, but there is no other way.

TO JOURNAL

- What three important things have you learned from previous relationships?
- What boundaries do you set in relationships to protect your well-being?
- What do people like about you? Are these the same things you like about yourself?

NINE

I AM THE TIN MAN

Within six months, I knew I had made a terrible mistake marrying Sam. He was possessive and emotionally abusive. I walked on eggshells at home. There were times I looked at him across the room and wondered *Who are you?* I felt I didn't know him and I certainly was not in love.

The strange sensation of him looking like my mother at our wedding dinner came back years later – I had married a man who represented how my mother made me feel; as a child, worthless and not valued. On some level, I had married my mother – or someone who would treat me as I thought I deserved. Born of low self-esteem.

Around this time, my diabetes got worse from all the stress in the marriage. One night I woke up and couldn't breathe. I had a stabbing pain in the middle of my back and my chest was tight. I got up and called Dr. Mirksy in the middle of the night. I got his service who woke him up.

I told him my symptoms and he said to me,

"This is what I want you to do. Do you have any ice cream at home?"

"Yes," I said.

"What kind?"

"Vanilla."

"Okay, I want you to take a big spoon and just eat one spoonful of vanilla ice cream."

I was confused by this but did as he advised and immediately felt better. I have never been able to figure out what he intuitively knew and how telling me to do that would relieve my symptoms.

The marriage continued to be stressful and I became more and more unhappy. I went to a therapist. Sam would accuse me of cheating on him every time I left the house. If we were out to dinner, he would accuse me of making eyes at other men. The therapist asked me why I didn't leave him. I said, 'I don't want to be alone."

She asked, "Aren't you alone now?"

I didn't have the strength or will to leave. My low self-esteem, unknown to me at the time, held me in place. I deserved to be unhappy. I deserved to be treated terribly in this relationship. I was the one causing him to act this way. It was my fault. I was terrified of life at that point, and it caused me to hunker down into an untenable marriage, come what may.

And what came was a monster bladder infection, which turned into a kidney infection. I had recurrent UTIs all the time but this was different. I called Dr. Mirsky's office and was told he was out of town, so I went to the nearest emergency room in Brooklyn.

I later found out this hospital was under federal investigation for incompetent care. At the time I was so sick I didn't know anything other than I hurt all over, had extreme exhaustion, nausea and terrible pain in my abdomen. After waiting in an open hallway on a gurney for five hours I was put into a room on one of the hospital floors.

It was crowded with three other patients, one of whom was handcuffed to the bed rails. A police officer sat on a chair outside the room.

I was clearly the sickest patient in the room and was unable to get up and use the bathroom by myself. A catheter was inserted. I didn't seem to have any doctor specifically assigned to me. I was too sick to care.

Four days went by and I got worse. They could not diagnose my problem – the nurses were hurried and curt and I just lay in this bed wondering what was happening to me. I could not even lift my arm. Sam came by at night after work, but was of no comfort. I found out later that he began to drink heavily again while I was sick. He could not handle the situation. He was not strong enough.

In the afternoon of the fourth day, I could feel myself desperately gripping physical reality. I was holding on as hard as I could, but I was so tired, so very tired. I felt trapped in the marriage, in fact, my life seemed a mess. There was nothing left for me to hold on to. I started to chant the sacred word HU that I learned about when I was 17 – that ancient name for God – HU – pronounced hue – but I was so tired it would only light up in my vision in two golden letters – H – U. I began to relax and let go of my worries and the fight to hold on. I sincerely said to God,

"If it's my time, I am ready to go."

I meant it. It was a relief to make that statement. I surrendered my feeling of holding on, gripping a physical reality that was slowly slipping away. I began to feel such peace.

Suddenly I heard a loud click. A movie started to play in front of my eyes — even though they were closed! I could see every detail of the scene in my mind's eye as this scene continued to play. It was accompanied by music. I could hear every note of the song being played, every detail of the scene as the vision continued. A movie projected on my mind's eye, playing on its own.

It was a scene from my favorite childhood movie *The Wizard of Oz.* The Tin Man has just been oiled after rusting in his body on the way to the Emerald City – and is so overjoyed with movement that he begins to dance and sing. His song was, *If I Only Had a Heart.* That's what he wanted from the wizard – a heart. I could feel the joy of his movement and feel the Tin Man's longing for a heart. Every note in the song made my heart tremble in recognition somehow. Even through my closed eyes, tears streamed down my face. I was the rusty Tin Man longing for love.

This inner movie faded and in the next moment, I was floating above my body – away from the feverish husk I'd been trapped in, holding on to so desperately. I felt such peace and calm. I was detaching from my physical body and reality – moving on energies of so much love and total acceptance - in me and of me. As I floated away from the body, I said to myself with deep wonderment, "So this is dying!"

There was no traveling in a tunnel toward a light, but there was light – bright white light everywhere. I was surrounded by it, enveloped in it, I was the light Itself. I felt so much love and compassion surrounding me from an invisible presence that was singular and divine. It was incredible and I was so far away from my life now. As I enjoyed this floating peace and freedom, I became aware of a sound like a low, rumbling, gentle hum. Then a sense of more than a few beings being present. They were talking in hushed tones. As soon as I realized this, the gentle rumbling hum stopped. I knew they had been talking about me. I could feel more than see them but the love and compassion was overpowering and complete – like every crack in my being was filled to the brim with pure spiritual love like a sparkling stream of light and sound.

A question came into my awareness telepathically.
Julia, do you want to go or do you want to stay?
I almost laughed it was so unexpected. I marveled at the question.

In a split second, I thought of my younger sister and her new baby. *I'll never get to meet that new Soul in our family.* It was a thought, not an answer. But it sealed the deal.

It was like a mighty vortex of wind came upon me and whooshed me through a moment of time: Boom! I was back in my body. Incredibly I had energy and a strong awareness of what to do next. I asked the nurse to hand me the phone. I called Dr. Mirsky.

He was back from his travels. I told him the situation. Without hesitation he carefully said:
"You will be strongly advised against this. But you *must* hire an ambulance and get to Mount Sinai hospital in Manhattan as soon as possible. Can you do that?"

"Yes," I replied.

So, with what little energy I had left, I called an ambulance service, and as Dr. Mirsky said, was strongly advised not to check out of the Brooklyn hospital. I signed the papers to go. Sam was a hovering presence but looked helpless. As they loaded me into the back of the ambulance, I lost all my energy again. I was again feeling so sick I could barely move. I closed my eyes and hoped that I could hold on a little longer and get to Dr. Mirsky.

The ambulance took off and turned on the siren. We went wailing over the Brooklyn Bridge into Manhattan toward Mt. Sinai Hospital. The ambulance siren was like the sirens I heard every day on the streets of New York. I would never again tune them out, but would say prayers of blessing for whomever was inside being rushed to a hospital. Because now I knew what it was like.

As the siren wailed and we sped forth, I had the most terrible thought – what have I done? Why did I choose to stay? It seemed like my life was darker than it was before and I longed for the earlier vision of the day — to feel that peace, love, compassion, and enveloping calm that I was deeply loved and cared for by a force greater than anything I had ever known. A very dark curtain came down on my heart. I was completely bereft.

Just at that moment the EMT who was sitting in the back with me put his hand on my arm and began to sing. It was an R&B song by Lionel Ritchie. He sang it as part lullaby and part hymn in the most beautiful baritone voice. It felt like an invitation to stay and trust all would be well.

Thanks for the times that you've given me
The memories are all in my mind
And now that we've come to the end of our rainbow
There's something I must say out loud

You're once, twice, three times a lady
And I love you
Yes, you're once, twice, three times a lady
And I love you
I love you

I felt like a divine force was singing these words to me, urging me to hold on. I was too tired to ask the EMT to keep singing and I was so afraid he would stop – it was keeping me in a cocoon of love. He continued to sing until we reached Mt. Sinai.

The siren was turned off and the ambulance stopped. The doors opened and they wheeled me out of the ambulance. This nameless, faceless EMT patted my arm as they rolled me away and said, "You're in good hands now." God bless him, wherever he is. I will never forget him.

The next hours were spent inserting tubes, taking X-rays, blood samples and getting settled in Intensive Care. I was exhausted beyond belief but felt a measure of comfort in this big hospital. My room was enclosed in glass and private. Dr. Mirsky arrived and his presence brought comfort. He was a tall man, with wild grey hair and rimless glasses which made his entire head look silver. He had an air of the befuddled professor, who was wildly intelligent and very personable. Like a favorite uncle. He assured me they were on my case.

My diagnosis: pneumonia, kidney and urinary infection, and e-coli sepsis. My blood had the infection and the pneumonia had gone undiagnosed for four days. I was in danger of going into septic shock and dying. My doctor talked to my parents through Sam and told them there was a 40% chance I would live through the night. He did not tell me this. With my diabetes complications, even at age 27, the sepsis was extremely dangerous even in a healthy person.

My mother flew out to be by my bedside. Each day was a chore to stay – my visions in the other hospital seemed so far away. I slept most of the days, didn't eat for weeks. Finally, after being fed intravenously, I could eat a spoonful of cooked peas. I was moved to a regular room. My roommate was a very elderly woman who screamed all night with a New York accent:

"Noice! Noice! I'm having a heart attack!"

After four more weeks, I was released to go home.

Back in our apartment, everything looked and felt different on a very deep level. I felt like a round peg in a square hole, like I didn't belong here on earth, that my home was somewhere else. Somewhere that was spiritually vibrant but so far away. The life I left was not the one I was returning to. Everything that interested me before seemed so trivial now. *Everything* seemed so trivial. People around me seemed like they were all sleepwalking. Newspapers and TV felt useless and lifeless. It was so much more than the marriage. I was not in this world, not grounded. I had landed on an alien planet and I missed my true home where I was deeply loved.

It took me a full year to come back fully to feeling like I was living a solid reality and was not some stranger in a strange land. It was like I had been taken apart atom by atom and put back together in an entirely different arrangement or design. I was me, but I no longer belonged on this earth. I had gone somewhere else and returned. I had fundamentally changed deep inside.

I had the powerful realization that for many years until that moment, I had no fear of death. Being so alive while out of my body obliterated any fear of death or dying. I knew myself to be an eternal being that had a temporary home in the body – for however long a lifespan would be. No, I had no fear of death. But what I realized is that I had a profound, deep-seated fear of living.

I was surrounded by good friends like Cheryl, who gave me love and support that I sorely needed to get grounded. My colleagues at work were also wonderful. But Sam was another story. The health crisis had unmoored him. He was drinking heavily all the time now and not hiding it. He was moody, aggressive, and more possessive than ever. Things came to a head four months later.

REFLECTIONS

I always knew there was some kind of invisible life behind some kind of veil in my imagination that was just out of reach. What secrets were held there? I read books, and watched movies, hoping for a glimpse. But it was not until I "died" in the hospital in Brooklyn, became the Tin Man in the Wizard of Oz and experienced an abundance of LOVE so overwhelming that the Light of it still brings pain to my inner eyes from the intensity. I was detached from this reality and fully existed, totally at peace, in another one where I was known, seen, loved, valued, and part of something so much greater than life here on earth. Nothing mattered but the wonder and awe I felt with the feeling of eternally being LOVED. A simple thought ended my sojourn, as so many simple thoughts begin new ones in our life every day.

This experience taught me so much about my body just being a vessel. A chariot for myself as Soul. I am Soul, I don't HAVE a Soul. That's who I am; you are and we are. Soul needs a rubber suit to live here – and mine had been through so much trauma already. It was now as if my atoms had been rearranged in mindset – and the true inner warrior in me was awakening. She was badass and determined, but had been allowing illusion to cloud her power. It was time for that to stop.

TO JOURNAL

- How do you feel about your body?
- Write a letter to your body. It's up to you to decide on the tone — is it a letter of congratulations, gratitude, an apology, a letter of complaint? When you reread it, does it feel like a letter to a friend?
- Is your inner warrior ready to come out? Why or why not?

TEN

DON'T ASK ME HOW I FEEL

I was working late for an important client and arrived home around 10 pm. This was about six months after I was released from the hospital and had healed from the infection.

Sam was drunk. As soon as I came through the door, he lunged at me and threw me against the wall – "Who have you been with?!" he demanded. Something about my experience in the hospital had awakened a sleeping warrior and she reacted – with some terror – but focused on survival.

I ran out the door and up the stairs to our neighbors' flat. They were a lovely couple with small children with whom we had socialized. I pounded on the door. Sam was too drunk to get up the stairs and went back inside and slammed the door to our apartment. My neighbors Drew and Annette didn't want to let me in. They had two toddlers and no idea what was going on. I said, "Please call the police!"

Annette called and Drew let me in. I was very upset but felt strength surging in me. The police came and soon it was 11:00 p.m. Sam had barricaded himself in the apartment below and would not come out. The police tried to talk him out but he wouldn't budge. They brought in a negotiator. Nothing. They ordered him out. He would not come out.

Meanwhile a female officer came to me and said she understood what I was going through, that she had been in an abusive relationship, too. It was little comfort, to be honest. But she was the only one who seemed to recognize I was traumatized.

At midnight a squad leader type came over to me and aggressively asked me exactly what Sam had done. He was still locked in the apartment and would not come out. This squad leader then accused me of not having any bruises, no ripped clothes or any injuries he could see. "So, what did he do exactly?!" he demanded to know.

I didn't have the energy to say: He has terrified me for the last 10 months with emotional abuse, physical abuse and treated me like a prisoner, accusing me of affairs every time I come home from work. He has belittled me, stalked me, harmed me on every level a woman is vulnerable and now has chased me out of my own home. That's what he had done. I am an emotional wreck, but that's changing tonight. And this squad leader was an extension of the male toxicity I had lived with in this short marriage.

My sixth sense was alive and I knew what he was getting at. It was midnight. Time for a shift change. The cops on the case now were being paid overtime because Sam would not come out and he was blaming me. I refused to talk to this toxic Squad Leader any longer.

At 2 a.m. the officers broke down the door and arrested him, asking me if I wanted to press charges. Yes, I did. They told me I had to go to the precinct to fill out papers and he'd be locked up until his court hearing in four days. Relief swept over me.

I stayed up that entire night putting his clothes in bags and ripping up every photo that was ever taken of us, including wedding photos. The marriage had lasted 10 months. Then I called my parents to tell them what happened. They were shocked of course, but I didn't have time to wallow and soak up their pity and sympathy. I was already feeling the energy shift in my life and I was going to ride that wave right out of this toxic situation.

By 6 a.m. it was light out so I took a taxi to the precinct where a large, kindly man took my information, called me "baby" and showed real concern for my welfare. It was so nice to be treated with care by a total stranger. I had isolated myself from friends and been encased in negativity, abuse, and desolation for months. Kind words from strangers can go a long way.

Things shifted quickly in the next days. I packed up my things, made arrangements to move in with Cheryl, and called the landlord to say I would not be renewing our lease, which was up that month. The bank had made an error with our joint account so they advised closing it. Unbeknownst to me, Sam had emptied it of all of our cash the week prior.

I got a new job in a part of the city where he could not find me. I started the new job the following week. I called a mover, taking my clothes and artwork and leaving everything else in the brownstone. I was DONE. Finito. Within a few weeks, I filed for divorce and Sam was served with divorce papers. It went uncontested and it was done. It was during this time I realized that I had never loved this man. I had agreed to the marriage so as not to be alone and to feel like I was loved. I had so much to learn!

Cheryl provided a safe haven for me. We'd been friends for so long it was like family. I felt safe. Eventually I moved out to a carriage house on the Hudson River — a calm, safe cottage on an estate. It was there that real loneliness and grief over a failed marriage and unknown future set in. I was 28 years old.

I found a therapist and started to go every week. I needed to know how I would end up with someone like Sam and how I could go that far without making better choices. I had a successful career, great friends, but utterly failed in relationships with men. Why? I always picked the wrong ones. Or I allowed the wrong ones into my space. Why?

I had to face things I had buried deep inside myself. I always thought I had a happy childhood – from the outside it would appear that way; my dad was a successful entrepreneur, we were all athletic, swam competitively, were cheerleaders, belonged to a country club and swam all summer. We took tropical vacations as a family in winter, lived in a big house in a nice neighborhood – really for that time, a typical Midwest middle class upbringing. However, appearances, as we know, are deceiving.

In reliving memories of my sister's death and experiences with my mother's rage, the flood gates opened and revealed a very wounded being inside. I had girded myself against feeling sorry all my life; and anytime I had shown feelings, my mother accused me of putting on an act. Cruel things would come out of her mouth that made no sense, like when our family dachshund Ginger died, and I cried. She said, "Why are you crying – you never liked the dog anyway."

When my first little brother was born, Dodi and Bamps came to visit for the first time. Bobby was the first grandson and bore Bamps' middle name in honor. I was 11 and I loved this new baby and loved to be around him.

Our grandparents left after the weekend to return home, a two-hour drive. Early the next morning, Bamps had a heart attack and died in Dodi's arms at home. We got the call around 6 a.m. At some point during that day, my mother said to me, "You made the last weekend of Bamps' life miserable! You wouldn't let him hold his own grandson! You helped him have a heart attack!"

I think about what must have been inside of her to make her say such things to a child. The loss of someone she dearly loved and respected, whose love she depended on, was now gone. Was she angry? Was she mentally unhinged? Was she reliving the loss of Nancy? As I have worked through the pain these comments brought on me as a child and into adulthood, I try to understand and accept the depth of her pain, how deeply wounded she was inside. I was an easy target. I wish she had received the support she needed in her life at that time. She had turned to the church, but she disappeared inside, and didn't come out for decades. The depth of her pain must have been monumental and that makes me very sad.

Nonetheless, comments were lobbed regularly, so I learned to shut my feelings down. Other times she would say very cruel things about other people and I'd feel like I knew more than she did, that those things weren't true. She said one time before the second baby brother was born, "I'm worried I won't have enough love to go around."

Even as a child I knew that love MULTIPLIED, it didn't get divided up. Words like these caused deep open wounds in my psyche, and I had to find a way to heal myself.

From age 14 to 16, I used recreational drugs to dull the pain but that didn't do anything but depress me more. Later, I turned to food. Though I didn't have anorexia or bulimia, I would binge eat to stuff down the feelings that wanted to come up. This went on for years.

I dreaded going home for holidays where my mother would make comments about my weight as if my value depended on that. I dreaded going unless I felt fit or good in my body – which was mostly never.

After the e-coli sepsis where I almost died, I lost so much weight I could barely stand, but my mother praised me for how I looked. The price I paid to get that way, almost dying from septic shock, totally escaped her notice. My mother probably exemplified women of her generation: never talk about anything below the surface, value looks above everything else. That was how you were judged in the wider world. It mattered so much what people thought about you.

One night while I was in therapy, I had a dream. I was pulling up what looked like huge turnips or garlic cloves from the ground with the help of a trusted presence. As we dug up these big bulbs, I saw they were filled with pus – infections that plagued my thinking and my life up to that point. It was a perfect symbol for how deeply they were buried and how big they were. Infectious thought and self-identity had planted them there since I was a child. I had ignored them until now. And the hard work was just beginning.

I began to hate the therapist for bringing up my mother in every session – she kept coming back to that subject. It exhausted me. Worse, she was constantly asking me, "How do you feel? How do you feel?" I hated that question.

There was one session where I sat in anger, not saying a word for the entire hour. But interestingly, I had shown up for the appointment. Her office was in a part of her home with a separate entrance for patients. It was always quiet at her house. But this appointment, her son was pounding on the piano on the other side of the wall, making discordant noise. He was around 11 and knew better. I was sure she put him up to it to get me to blow up in anger, but I remained silent and bottled up. Her ploy didn't work.

I left after the silent hour was up – I was so sick of talking about my mother and how I felt. Her question, "How do you feel, how do you feel, how do you feel?" kept ringing in my ears. On the drive home through a dark wooded area, I pulled the car over and screamed what was bubbling up from deep inside: MY FEELINGS DON'T FUCKING MATTER!

The crux of the matter was that not only did my feelings not matter, but I didn't matter. I buried these feelings deeply so that no one, even myself, could not discern what they were. The feelings that allowed me to walk into a toxic relationship with a man like Sam – and then marry him – were not around to warn and protect me. He aligned with my low opinion of myself – men like that saw women like me a mile away. They know we are weak, and easy prey to a controlling, angry toxicity. They know the relationship will be unbalanced in their favor. We will do anything to keep them happy, all at the expense of our own happiness. They matter more than we do – we are nothing, worthless, we deserve to be treated like shit. My god, where do these ideas come from? They were so hidden from my conscious mind – I had no idea what a low opinion I had of myself. I had no boundaries, no protective sense of what was good for me in a relationship.

Louis, who adored and cherished me, I pushed away constantly. The unknowing, unrealized feeling part of me knew I was NOT worth it. I was annoyed he would be so loving and caring to me. I was nothing. That he reminded me constantly that I was something, cherished and adored pissed me off. It did not align with my deepest feelings about myself. I had hidden those feelings since they began to bloom in childhood. I tucked them so far down in my psyche among the other wounds that I had no idea – none at all — that they were steering me into volatile relationships with men. I simply did not know. Until that night on the road, driving home from the therapist, angry as hell at her for asking me how I felt. My feelings until that moment were worthless, not worthy of discussion or reflection. They didn't matter. I didn't matter.

A flash of insight revealed the darkness I had lived in so deep down that I could not see it. It was time to heal. My body had taken on the sense of devastation in my life during the episode with the sepsis infection. To the point where I was willing myself to just go. Leave this life. My body had already seen so much trauma.

I didn't fear death.

No, I feared life.

I feared living fully in the light of my true potential. As the warrior woman emerged from my inner shadows, I would alternately be feeling strong and free and also terrified. My true potential was becoming visible. Was that what I was here for?

REFLECTIONS

Thus began the seeds of knowing how to manage my life and how to find happiness within: first, how to sweep out the demons and dust devils inside, and find my worth.

Our thoughts, desires and emotions hold tremendous energy. Whether they are unconscious or conscious they exist as an exacting blueprint that determines our outer reality. Like a broadcasting tower we send out vibrations all the time and the Universe, God energy, or whatever one identifies as what Yoda calls "the Force" returns this to you in hard atoms. It's a plastic universe molded by our thoughts – what we think about constantly deep down, we believe.

Our bodies are the battleground on which we can see what lies hidden beneath the surface. Until you look there, self-sabotage, inability to commit to a program or nutrition plan, lack of motivation and no willpower will be blamed for one's failure to "get in shape." It's beyond all those excuses. It's in the thoughts we think, what we believe about ourselves.

We think it's about weight loss. But that only addresses the body, which is governed by two more turning wheels in our being: mindset and spirit. We keep throwing diets at the body and it never is sustainable. Why? We don't address mindset and "spirit set" – we ignore the richest parts of who we are.

TO JOURNAL

- Do you believe you deserve to be healthy, strong, lean, and beautiful? If yes, why, if no, why not?
- What kind of self-talk do you live with every day?
- How differently do you speak to yourself than you would your very best friend?

ELEVEN

THE MASK CAME OFF

My mother was born in 1934 and was not planned. She had three older brothers who doted on her but there was at least 15 years between her and the youngest brother – the oldest was 18. Her father was a wonderful man who carved little characters out of wood, hand-fed squirrels in their backyard and loved his dogs. He seemed gentle and caring with a wicked sense of humor. But he was also an alcoholic – so who knows what that created in my mother's life. In all the pictures we have of her from age three to around 16 she looks angry – as if she can't get away from her old parents soon enough.

Yet she was a beauty and she married her best friend Nancy's brother, my dad, just six months after meeting him.

She left college to marry and embarked on the 1950's pinnacle for women according to society: motherhood and becoming a housewife. She missed the boat on all the emancipation that women demanded in the 1960's; by the time she was 27 she had four children under the age of 6. It was not what she had planned for her life – she wanted a college education and had started on one, then my dad came along and they fell in love.

As a small child, I noticed that she was frustrated and angry. She lost her temper easily and had no patience for what it took to raise four girls under the age of six. It was so hard for her. She had dreams that went unrealized. She suffered from a great loss within herself.

When I was 8, my parents got a babysitter and said they were meeting with our church pastor for the evening. When they arrived home, they sat us all down – Nancy, who was 5 at the time had been in the hospital, but we weren't told why. She was third in a line-up of girls, just after me. I was the second oldest.

My parents looked very serious and began to explain that Nancy was sick and needed an operation – I remember the square vinyl TV cushion I sat on by the brick fireplace in the family room. I had never seen my parents so seriously addressing us as parents. Their demeanor alarmed me. I interrupted, blurting – "Is she going to...."

I didn't get the word out, before my mother cut me off and said forcefully, "No, we are not going to lose her!"

During a year of painful trips to the hospital and missing out on birthdays, holidays, and simple days, our dear Nancy battled the sarcoma cancer that kept growing inside her tiny abdomen. They took the tumor out twice and it came back twice.

In the 1960s the medical field would do anything to save the life of a child – unlike today, where the beloved child is allowed to return home for comfort and palliative care in their final months.

My mother would take Nancy to the emergency room, my dad would be on a business trip, and she'd make sure Nancy was in a room being cared for, then drive home, pulling the maroon station wagon into the garage, getting out and collapsing on the floor in sobs. She would wipe away tears as soon as she saw us looking. It must have been so devastating and awful for her.

My dad would take Nancy on long drives in his light blue Mustang and they would sing songs from the musical *West Side Story*. Her favorite was *I'm So Pretty*. Her favorite TV show was *Lost in Space* and I like to think I was her favorite sister – being only three years apart. She looked up to me and had the sweetest temperament. Her hair was dark and the other three of us were blonde, so she always stood out. She had such grace at such a young age – maybe she knew she was not long for this world. Her middle name was Adore – a combination of my two grandmother's names – Alice and Dorothy. She was named after Nancy, my mom's best friend from childhood and now her sister-in-law.

From age 5 to 6, Nancy wasted away to nothing. Her huge brown eyes shone with intelligence, humor, and love. How is that possible I think to this day that at the end of her life she exudeed such grace and beauty? She was nonchalant about what she faced – clearly, she didn't know what was in store, nor did she seem to care. She was just herself, an incredibly brightly lit child suffering from a devastating cancer who always faced each day with joy.

On my first day of fourth grade, I came home for lunch. The house was quiet. I heard my mother softly call me upstairs. She was sitting on the edge of the bed in the master bedroom, with a tissue in her hand. Her nose was red. Her eyes were red. She had been crying. She told me without preamble,

"Nancy's with God."

Stunned and unbelieving, it sunk in. As I started to weep, she said Nancy's last words were, "Where are the girls?" – meaning her sisters.

I had the overwhelming need to be by myself. I just wanted to be alone. Still softly crying, I went to my room where I had a walk-in closet. I sat down in there, turned on the light and closed the door. I felt desolate, empty, and completely shattered. But on another level, I accepted this reality and didn't fight the blow it gave me. I just sat with it. I was nine years old.

I looked up at the clothes hanging above me and thought with disgust that this very morning, my very first day of fourth grade, I had been so concerned with what I wore to school! While my little sister was dying! The futility of it in the face of this loss staggered me. I was selfish, self-centered, and unfeeling just like my mother told me I was. The guilt was unbelievable and weighed heavily on my small shoulders. My tears were not only for the loss of my beloved sister, but for the horrible guilt and regret I now carried.

My father had not been at the hospital when Nancy passed and had rushed home to us. When he entered, he crouched down and gathered his three daughters into his arms and hugged us all at once saying, "Always see Nancy growing up in your minds." I remember being in the corner of the family room when he did this, looking out at the brick fireplace where we'd first heard Nancy was sick one year before. My father's strength and resolve were comforting and so were his tears.

I took what he said to heart, and every year on her birthday, March 3, I see the beautiful Soul she was who took form for only a short while. I have seen her grow up in my mind, following in age three years behind me. My father's wise words made sense to me year after year on Nancy's birthday – it's a sacred ritual to see her growing up in my imagination. My younger sister was too little to comprehend what was happening; my brothers were not born yet, and my older sister processed it differently than I did. But every year on March 3, I either called or wrote my parents to say how much I loved and remembered Nancy. She was a major catalyst for me to begin questioning my own reason for being alive, and set me on a spiritual search for answers to life's deepest questions.

Our parents decided it would be best if we girls did not attend the memorial service for Nancy. We stayed home with a babysitter. Afterward, close family and friends were at the house. From that day forward, my grandma Ritchey, my Mom's mom had only one picture in her bedroom: that of Nancy. She could see it every night before she lay down to sleep. My grandmother Dodi was present, and so was my Aunt Nancy, who could not contain her tears.

At the round game table in the living room with low chairs next to the fireplace, I watched my mother in her grief. She was defeated, she had surrendered, she was spent, and she was crying softly — weeping with deep, genuine emotion. I had never seen her look so vulnerable. So beautiful. Her mask was off, and there she was in all her beauty. I only wanted to care for her in her grief. Her surrender was clear as day. I was nine years old but felt like I was 99 because of what I could perceive in her. It made me love her deeply. I saw her. I was overcome with tenderness for my mother who had caused me so much emotional pain.

That night Nancy's favorite TV show was on: *Lost in Space*. My dad remarked on this and when he said, "The episode tonight is called *Wishing on a Star,*" he broke down in tears. We all sat on the family room couches facing the TV — my parents and three girls, playing out a family ritual of TV watching that gave comfort, but also was a harsh reality. Nancy was not with us.

I felt a deep sense of caring for my mother and wanted to make her feel better. But as the months wore on, she withdrew into a haze of rigidity and completely shut down emotionally. Her mask came on and was held in place by impossible grief. She had held emotions in check before, but now she was robotic. Church became her refuge and she hid behind the dogma as if it would shield her from the pain.

Years later she told me acquaintances would avoid her in the grocery store, thinking that cancer was contagious; she felt more alone than ever. It took her decades to lift the lid on that period of time and share snippets of what she had experienced and the trauma that was heaped on her during and after Nancy's death. Her self-care involved getting busy and wrapped up in the church. She became the office manager and spent hours helping the head pastor. Like most women she was an expert multi-tasker, incredibly organized, and could focus on a task like a laser beam. All else disappeared. In fact, that's what it felt like after Nancy died. My mother completely disappeared – she was no longer emotionally connected to our day-to-day concerns as children.

When I was in my 30's, my mother shared the poignant moment that Nancy passed away. If anything, my mother had a deep sensitivity and sense of the invisible side of life that was enveloped in Christian practices. We were probably more alike than different and that's one reason we had a hard time – we mirrored each other's weaknesses to one another.

My mother had been at Nancy's bedside in the hospital. Right before Nancy took her last breath, my mother said she heard the fluttering of wings as if she had come upon a flock of large birds. She said it was unmistakable – and then my mother felt herself go "somewhere" and come back – and Nancy was gone. She told me she had the same "going somewhere and coming back" each time she gave birth to her children.

I understood that to mean she journeyed to the invisible side of life – where Soul comes and goes in birth and in death – and that there is the eternal part of us that travels these realities we call life. My mother and I were more alike than different.

As I got older, I came to understand all the pain my mother experienced in losing Nancy and how she was not equipped to deal with life's blows in a way that didn't affect her children. From the age of nine to 14, I didn't have a mother – emotionally she was absent and I learned to take care of myself. I became a survivor. I would survive by myself at all costs. While she was trying to survive by herself.

REFLECTIONS

It was an actual gift to be made strong through hard experience. My mother was a catalyst. I was given the tools I needed to survive what was to come later in my life. We all have this strength inside of us that doesn't get tested or revealed until things get really tough. We look at it as a terrible thing, but it's really revealing the warrior we are inside, the eternal being we are now and forever. The part of us that deeply understands life and why we are here – and who we truly are. It's there. The hard experiences will bring it out. That's the silver lining of life's pain.

It's taken me years to use this awareness and strength to overcome unhealthy habits, ways of thinking, and build self-esteem. Each little step, each boundary set around toxic situations and people, each time I said "No," or honored my feelings, I built self-trust. It feels empowering to take care of yourself.

TO JOURNAL

- What relationships in your life were the most difficult but taught you the most? How did this happen?
- Complete this sentence and then keep writing: "I owe an apology to ____"
- Surrealist artist Salvador Dalí once said: "Have no fear of perfection — you'll never reach it." How does that sentence make you feel?

TWELVE
NO ONE UNDERSTANDS BUT YOU

In my thirties, my medical history made the odds of me surviving beyond the age of 40 a slim possibility. Childhood diabetes eventually brought on all the diabetes complications: neuropathy, retinopathy, heart disease, and then kidneys failing. It started in my early 20's.

There were other obstacles I needed to overcome and those took decades. Feelings of unworthiness, lack of self-esteem, a denial of my emotions. There were reasons for this, experiences that imprinted false knowledge on my vulnerable child-heart.

There were years of trying to fill the hole inside and discovering that nothing out here would do it. But the seeking and striving for an answer never stopped despite the futility of my searching. Why were my relationships with men always with those who ultimately didn't treat me well? Why was I so intent on losing weight and never finding a permanent solution? Why was I so unhappy in my own skin?

My physical body wore the mark of my striving as I stuffed down feelings with food, got disgusted with my lumpy thighs and went whole-hog into a weight loss program — many times. My unhappiness did not abate when I lost weight, it just made me a skinnier version of the same unhappy person. And, for good measure, it always returned with more pounds.

Food is a dangerous weapon if we use it that way. We have to eat to live – but often we eat to assuage emotional trauma, hidden feelings, anxiety, and stress. It's an awkward dance of control and lack of control, discipline and say to hell with it. Our relationship with food plays out in our insecurities in our relationships — and exposes our relationship with ourselves.

Do you love yourself? Or do you constantly hear negative self-talk in your head toward yourself? I hate my stomach, thighs, arms, dowager hump, batwings, back fat – the self-loathing is like poison.

We are bundled energies on physical, emotional, mental and spiritual levels. Our thoughts carry that energy through us and into the world. The Universe responds to our thoughts, because we are co-creators of our life – and fills the mold we create with those thoughts with manifested reality. There is a time lapse despite the speed of thought, so often we don't make the connection. But whatever you believe and hold deep down to be true will become your reality. The Universe simply responds to your thought frequency and brings you what you most think about. Worry about money? Your looks? Getting old? Be careful with your thoughts – they carry the truth of your life into being.

When you change your thought patterns to positive, goal oriented, self-loving ones, it can take a long time for them to manifest, especially if you haven't been in that practice for years. But hold onto it and it will happen.

I decided at age 62 that I was running out of time. I felt compelled to do something out of complete joy and gratitude to be alive. I had to start to honor the body I was in and celebrate that it had gone through so much and was still working well. I wanted to be strong, vital, healthy, and incredibly fit – and found my way to that goal over a two-year period by day-in and day-out dedication to the ideal in my heart and mind of who I wanted to be.

The first time I picked up a dumbbell to lift weights I was "her" – the strong fit, healthy woman I became within two years outwardly. In that split second of accepting that as my reality, I was her. It would just take time for it to manifest out here.

Along the way I found a strength inside that was always there, but now was fueled by deep gratitude to be alive. My structure of nutrition and training everyday built on and, on each day. It became a platform from which my view of life changed drastically from passive acceptance to galvanized energy to transform. I transformed on the inside in ways that surprised me, and this was much more powerful than the outer transformation. Because it's where all true transformation comes from – the inside.

A goal like weight loss is shallow and unsustainable and only accounts for an outer effect. I went for a bigger goal, a more expansive outcome of optimal health, strength, and vitality. Weight loss was a side effect.

During all those years before, when body disgust would spur me to go on another diet, the deprivation of food felt worthwhile – it was a way of punishing myself for being undisciplined about my eating. It was never sustainable.

For years and years, I was disciplined about food – as a young diabetic, I had to be. My relationship with food was complicated. I needed it to live but weaponized it or made it my enemy. It was the cause of all my diabetes complications in the way that it affected my blood sugars.

Nothing I did would balance my blood sugars, as my case was "brittle" – and my body was sensitive to everything that could interfere with proper insulin absorption. The complications of the disease took hold by age 24 starting with proliferative retinopathy. The small blood vessels in my eyes leaked blood into my retina. It was the beginning of diabetic blindness.

In addition to the health challenges, and food issues there were unresolved emotional issues surfacing in my life in my early 20's.

I often had a feeling in the "back of my mind" of what "they" would think if I did something bold and risky. Or if "they" would notice I was out of shape. Would "they" notice the good, bad, or ugly in my life?

This "they" was always in the background: judging, criticizing and non-accepting. It was like a blurred-out crowd of faceless, nameless people watching my every move. Ready to disapprove and reject me. They followed me everywhere.

The "they" were me, of course.

My mom, a frustrated wife of the 1960's who missed the boat on emancipation, had dreams that went unrealized. Though my dad was an amazing provider and loving father and husband, my mom was a very angry person. I thought of her as a rage-aholic. Often, I was criticized, judged, disapproved of and worst of all my feelings were constantly negated. Emotional vulnerability was terrifying to her so she shut down and wanted to shut me down, too.

People out in the world wore the face of my mother: judgmental and non-accepting. I got into relationships with men who reinforced this false belief. Even during the wedding dinner with Sam and my parents, I saw the "they" on his face. It was the same face my mom wore. This "they" presence stalked me.

To uproot this took work. And my mom, God love her, did her best. I honor the warrior in her that drove her to survive during unspeakable loss. She didn't just lose a child, she had to watch a beloved child suffer – suffer for a year, knowing there was nothing she could do to alleviate the pain. I heard her say once, during Nancy's illness, "I wish it were me."

Due to the family dysfunction, I left the tribe of home early to become an adventurer. So, it was a gift to have that kind of mother. It made me strong – stronger than I ever would have been – and I needed that to survive what life was going to hand me going forward.

Once I could remove "they," all bets were off. I felt empowered and free to do what I wanted. Self-sabotage disappeared as I aged. My mom, though it was incredibly painful for her, provided a crucible to make me strong. She didn't even know it. God bless her.

I needed all these experiences to get to the point I am today in taking care of my body, mind, and soul. The hardest experiences were the richest. Today, I don't lay blame anywhere, but accept each bruise and wound as a fresh opportunity for learning more about life, myself, and how to live purposefully.

My mother had her own path carved through the crucible of pain – and she was without the support from other women she desperately needed. She was caught between a 1950's housewife and the emancipated 1960's, and was unable to realize her dreams in life. She had plans, she was an incredible writer and organizer, and much of her anger and frustration must have come from not having agency to really go after her dreams of education and a career.

Over the decades, she got grandchildren, which began to soften her. She still lacked emotional balance and tried to control situations that were not hers to control, but she had a loving heart that longed to give. She was not sure how, because being vulnerable was not safe for her. She put her love into making beautiful, handmade colorful quilts for all her family. She knitted and crocheted little hats for premature infants at the hospital, since premature triplets had been born to one of my siblings. One tiny beloved baby passed away after two weeks, another was disabled with cerebral palsy – and so she had a very soft spot for preemies.

Taking care of my dad, who developed diabetes in his '50s, was her day-to-day focus for years. He was a virile man in his younger years but the diabetes, COPD, arthritis, and other ailments debilitated him as he aged into his 80s. She was his nurse and caregiver for more than 20 intense years.

As his episodes of falling and terrible coughing fits from the COPD continued, dementia started to show. She was a small woman and could not risk my dad falling and not being able to help him get up, and there were plenty of 911 calls. So, it was decided he should enter a senior care home with 24-hour nursing.

My husband of 30 plus years, Paul, and my dad had become great friends over the years since getting married in

1989. They were golfing buddies, sports fans together, and people-loving men who could talk to anyone. They were alike in so many ways. In Paul, I had married a man like the father I adored.

We were living in Saudi Arabia when my brother called to say my father had passed. My reaction came from my heart, up through my chest and into my throat, in one long protracted wail of grief. It was literally a cry of pain. I was so far away from him when he died, which felt awful. Within six hours we were on a plane to be with my family in the U.S.

Three years later, my brother, Bob called in October 2019 to say my mom had gone into the ER and they'd done a cardiac catheterization which showed advanced heart disease. She was 85 and there was no way to put in a stent or do a bypass. Anyway, she would have refused it. The doctors recommended palliative care for her remaining time. Her greatest fear was that she would be a burden to any of us and she was fiercely independent. Decisions were made with her doctor and my siblings and we set her up in a lovely hospice-care facility. She never made it back to her own home after the ER visit. Her hospice room opened onto a private garden. It was a quiet peaceful environment with French doors that opened to colorful autumn leaves, sunshine, and warm days.

All my siblings, their spouses and the grandkids visited her there over the succeeding three weeks. Paul and I drove from Savannah to Indianapolis – 14 hours each way, with the dogs in the back.

The doctors had her on morphine and were giving her breathing treatments to ease her lack of oxygen and her feeling of suffocating. The morphine brought out the shine in her. She reveled in all of us surrounding her bed each day, listening to her recite spiritual poems and enjoying classical music. The mask was off and laid aside. There was nothing left to fight anymore. As she lay in her hospice bed, the sunlight would come in and bathe her in gold. She never looked more beautiful. When her mask was off, she was incredibly radiant.

In a raspy voice, she recited this poem several times with her eyes closed:

God hath not promised skies always blue,
Flower-strewn pathways all our lives through;
God hath not promised sun without rain,
Joy without sorrow, peace without pain.
But God hath promised strength for the day,
Rest for the labor, light for the way,
Grace for the trials, help from above,
Unfailing sympathy, undying love.

Near the end, one granddaughter came to her bedside and could not contain her tears. Her nose got stuffed up and she was sniffling and quietly sobbing. My mother looked at her and said, "Honey do you have a cold?" She couldn't recognize the grief. Perhaps it was the morphine. I laughed with Paul later, she just wasn't an emotional woman, but she could shed tears at a Hallmark card commercial on TV.

We took turns spending the night with her. No one wanted her to be alone at night, despite the hospice care being excellent. The last week, I was the one who slept by her bed to make sure if she woke up, I could attend to her needs, call the nurse, get her what she wanted. I thought of all the times she was at my bedside during my brushes with death. My nine-year-old self was finally able to care for the vulnerable soul who now stood on the threshold of leaving this life.

More than 50 years later. It felt like a circle was beautifully completed.

During the last week, she said with wonderment, "I'm looking forward to seeing what heaven is like." She was excited and at peace, ready for her transition.

Once when no one was around – she looked me in the eyes and said, "When is it going to happen?"

I said, "Mom, just allow it to come naturally, it will happen when you stop looking for it." My own experiences with near death and dying gave me a special view of this sacred time. She knew it, though had never acknowledged it.

"No one understands but you," she said.

"I know, Mom."

This was light years away from our decades earlier conversations about anything spiritual. When I was 17, I was a true seeker, reading anything I could get my hands on – anything that was not in the Christian tradition I grew up with. I felt it had not answered my questions about life or death, and that my mother was not a good role model for it. Not with her split personality of at church/at home. Of course, I was seeing through young eyes. Nonetheless, I turned from that tradition just at a time when she felt it her mission in life to make sure all her children accepted Christ as savior. Or we'd go to hell.

My interest in other sacred teachings scared and angered her. She felt everything was a cult and I was a cult member. I felt religious persecution by my own mother for having ideas that were spiritually searching and expansive. They did not fit neatly into her narrow view of religion.

Maybe this was where we were alike. My mother always had a sixth sense, was attuned to the spiritual side of life in a way that worked for her, but my way was foreign yet similar. I acknowledged things that she did not want to address.

All those years she must have watched me go through my medical challenges and over hurdles of life and death, and saw my strength come from *somewhere*. Maybe she saw it as the same divine source she looked to in her final hours. Because when she looked at me and said "You are the only one who understands," I knew that she knew. She knew that we were in agreement spiritually, finally. That I knew her transition was a spiritual event of the greatest magnitude. And that ultimately love was the glue between us. It had been all along.

We had to return home and Paul and I went to see her before driving off, not knowing if this was the last time. Would I see her again or would she would pass in the next week?

Paul leaned over and poured the most loving words into my mother's ears that I have ever heard uttered. This man, my tall, green-eyed love, gave my mother all the love that I was unable to really express in a way that came purely from his heart, no strings. I can't tell you exactly what his words were but they were like a devotional prayer to the sanctity of her life lived and how honored he was to know her — this beautiful soul.

I knelt by her bed and held her hand.
"Mom I love you so much, thank you for everything." I just kept repeating those words and she said, "I love you too."

I kissed her; then we left and drove 14 hours back home to Savannah.

But the next weekend she was still alive and we returned.

I spent the night with her again. It was clear she was very close to leaving. I didn't sleep much that night and was hyper-aware of her every move. She was in such a deep state. We had said what needed to be said the last time so this was just to hold her hand and be there.

In the morning I could tell she was no longer present in her body. She was still breathing but she was not there. I called my brother and younger sister – the two who were really her favorites, if truth be told.

I was never affected by that – I marveled at how my younger sister adored my mother; it was so clear during her time in hospice. At one point my sister looked at our mother as she slept – and said to me, "GOD! I love her so much!"

I was deeply touched and in awe of the love she felt for a mother for whom I could not express that depth of love. Of course, I loved her, but it was a hard-earned love. I had to heal my past and see her as a woman struggling to live life when it was falling apart around her. We spoke completely different love languages.

I told my brother on the phone that mom was still breathing, but she was gone. Within fifteen minutes both he and my younger sister were at her bedside. I knew she was not going to open her eyes again, so I told Paul we needed to pack up and think about another 14-hour drive.

We left the hospice and returned to where we were staying. As we were packing up, my brother texted – Mom's breathing has changed. Please come quickly.

We drove as fast as we could back to the hospice and as I entered the room, both my brother and sister were on either side of mom holding her hand. She had just taken her last breath in the presence of the two children she adored. It was as if she allowed me to go in peace and waited for those two to be with her. I was deeply moved and happy for her.

A circle had closed. Completed itself. Of all the trauma and pain growing up, and all the challenges it gave me to be her daughter, there was only one thing left at the end. One thing only that mattered. Love.

REFLECTIONS

To be at the deathbed of a loved one can be traumatizing or enlightening. Since my own brushes with death, I have a more detached view of the body – and how it is a chariot for who we are as a living Soul – it's our vehicle to get around in the world. It's not who we really are – it's just our vehicle. My awareness was I was never afraid of dying or death, but very afraid of living. Living fully and fearlessly! Not fearlessly in high-risk behavior, which was in my past, but being willing to look life square in the eye and say: LET'S GO! I'm ready to take you on and realize my dreams as reality!

Our bodies become the battleground for the internal wars we have within ourselves starting (for me) in adolescence. Not taking care of it, ignoring its needs, abusing it through drugs and alcohol, or lack of proper nutrition. It's amazing it can last for so many decades before it begins to break down.

We make decisions based on what "they" will think – this same nameless, faceless group of people who live in our heads – all the criticism, negativity, confidence killers we have encountered in our life. They seem real and constantly vigilant about everything we do. We watch our step so as not to invite more criticism, censure, and disappointment.

And who are "they?" Our own selves, of course. Us. Self-sabotage ensues from this invisible force we have set up. We are in a self-made prison.

It's never too late to turn things around. In body, mind or spirit.

The body is always seeking balance, healing, and optimal functioning – on its own as a living organism – as a chariot for the Soul. Answering that call of balance is the greatest self-gift we can give. That balance comes from a deeper part of who we are. The wheels that turn in body, mind, and spirit want to turn in tandem.

The transitory nature of life, and our limited time here was what really helped me begin my fitness journey at age 62. I knew I didn't have any more time to mess around with my health. The time was now.

TO JOURNAL

- Who judges you most harshly? Has it caused you to be hard on yourself?
- Have you weaponized food to self-punish or distract from feelings?
- Imagine a world where you could do everything you like without being judged by the people around you. Would anything change in your life?

THIRTEEN

SEA GREEN EYES

In 1988, seven months after my divorce to Sam was finalized, I attended a conference in Houston, Texas with some friends. We wore our name tags out for dinner and waited at the Benihana Restaurant for a table. I was sitting facing the door, in the dark lobby. Suddenly the door opened and a very tall man appeared in silhouette with some friends. I could barely make out that he had on a name tag like ours. When he stepped into the dim light an electric shock went up my spine and I wanted to blurt out, incredulously and joyously at the same time, "WHAT ARE YOU DOING HERE?!"

I had never seen him before in my life.

It was like being in a remote corner of the world, turning a corner and seeing your best friend from childhood or lifetimes ago.

I noted his eyes – the color of a calm sea in pale green, and the three-button blue Henley shirt he wore and the blond color of his hair and his sharp, gracious nose. He and his friends were attending the same conference we were. We invited them to sit with us at a hibachi table. One of my friends was sitting between him and me. I could not get enough of him – I blathered on and on asking him where he was from (Iowa) how he liked the conference (very much) and on and on.

As we completed dinner the feeling left me like a glowing coal that had flamed and then gone out. We all went back to our respective hotels. I kept running into him at the conference and we stole a moment here and there to sit in the lobby and chat. I was a city girl, and here was this goofy guy from Iowa – kind and sweet, but goofy. Corny even. I decided he was a good guy and we became friends.

He showed me a picture of his 11-year-old daughter, but I didn't ask about her mother. It was none of my business. I didn't tell him I'd divorced the previous March. It was not going to go that way – romantic, that is. I was not looking for a partner – at all.

Over the course of the next year, he wrote me letters and I would write back. It was clear now that he and his wife were separated and getting a divorce. I didn't ask a lot of questions because I was not interested in anything other than a friendship. Besides, he was not my type. I was not attracted to him "that way."

His letters were kind and sweet and interested in my life. When I had more laser eye surgery in NYC for retinopathy, he sent me a gift of a blooming plant to cheer me up. I thought what a sweet friend he was. Then he suggested I should come to Iowa for a visit. That stopped me cold – I was not going to go visit this new friend all the way in Iowa, a single man in his 30s, me single, just turned 30, and have it be an issue where I slept. I did not want that kind of pressure or relationship but he was such a gentleman he never suggested to go in that direction.

To get him off the topic, I blithely said one time, "Well, you should come visit NYC after the conference in Washington," thinking he'd never take me up on it. It was just a nicety. But he called one day in the summer and said, "Hey I'm getting my tickets for Washington."

I said "Yeah? Great!"

Silence.

"You said to come visit NYC sometime and I thought maybe I could ride the train back with you after the conference in DC."

Oh shit. Say something, Julia.

"Um, yeah! Okay, sure! That would be great."

Shit shit shit.

After we hung up, I invited my younger brother to come and visit me the exact same weekend so that there would be an extra male presence in the house and I would not feel put upon. I trusted my new friend but I was not ready for any kind of relationship. Just a little extra insurance against awkwardness.

We met at the conference and he later took the train to NYC with me with my brother in tow. On the train ride to NYC, we looked off to the right and there were fireworks in the sky. It almost escaped my notice and didn't seem unusual.

Finally, we arrived at my Hudson River carriage house. He got the guest room and my brother slept on the floor in the living room. I told him I needed him there just to deflect any weirdness if it happened. My brother understood. The same dear brother who was with me when the priest who married me to Sam didn't recognize us.

My tall friend with the green eyes was a bit subdued that weekend after the conference and seemed very contemplative and quiet. He pulled out some photos after dinner one night – of him when he was a little boy – I took a glance and said, "So cute!" And handed it right back.

God, Julia, get a clue. But I was clueless. I held him at arm's length all weekend and was my usual self – meaning sometimes grumpy and impatient. I made no special attempt to glamourize myself for the male gaze. I was used to dressing and acting in ways that would attract male attention but my first marriage cured me of that and I was just . . . well, I was just me.

In all my Julia –ness, which can be charming or not. Depending on my health situation at the time.

At the end of the weekend, as he waited for the airport bus to pick him up, he looked sad. I thought he must be thinking about his divorce. I knew it would finalize in a month. We said good-bye and did a friendly kiss. I worried he was brooding about his ex-wife. After all, he was by now a dear friend.

That was in August. In October we would see each other again in Atlanta for another conference. The offers to visit Iowa stopped, which was fine with me.

I got to the Atlanta hotel on Friday and settled in the room with my friend Cindy. We were up at midnight talking when I was overwhelmed with the feeling that I would be alone the rest of my life and never meet anyone to love.

My friend listened with an open heart and I cried and cried saying how alone I felt.

"I have so much love to give and no one in my life to give it to. I guess I'll just be an old maid. I'm never going to meet anyone." Cindy assured me that would probably not be the case, but I was convinced and despondent.

At that moment our room phone rang. Cindy answered. It was my tall green-eyed friend. She handed me the phone.

"He wants to talk to you. "

"How are you?" I said.

"Hi! What are you doing right now? "

"Right now?"

"Yeah. "

"Cindy and I are just talking." (And I'm crying my eyes out because I have no one in my life to love and to love me.)

"Do you want to come down and ride the elevators?" So goofy Iowa of him – riding the outside elevators of the hotel for fun.

"Sure." It would get my mind off my troubles.

I said to Cindy, "He wants us to come down and ride the elevators! Let's go."

Even though it was midnight, I was not up for sleeping. I needed diversion. Cindy and I took the elevator down to the lobby.

When the doors opened in the lobby and I saw him standing there, he looked shocked for a moment but recovered, smiled, and greeted both of us.

We spent the next hours riding the elevators, glass enclosures that whooshed up and down the outside of the high-rise hotel with a view of the Atlanta skyline. At one point we were looking out over the skyline and we saw fireworks.

Again. Like on the train from Washington to NYC. We got a bite to eat, after meeting more friends – everyone seemed nocturnal! Cindy and I prepared to leave and I said, "I'll see you tomorrow at the conference."

The oddest thing happened when we got back to our room at 2:00 AM and I laid my head down to go to sleep. I could swear that I felt his head on the pillow next to mine. Weird! I rolled over and fell asleep.

The next morning, we arranged to sit together for the final keynote talk. I was tired from the night before, being out so late. At some point during the talk, I fell asleep and my head fell onto his shoulder. I only awoke when the applause started for the keynote speaker.

As I opened my eyes, it was like coming out of a dream — or going into one – because without a shred of doubt the feeling in my heart was:
Oh MY GOD! I am IN LOVE with this man!!

I was so startled I could barely move – I felt like a secret had been withheld from me and now here it was in full reckoning. No one told me! How did this happen? It was as if in falling asleep I was taken to a place and the scales were removed from my heart so I could actually see what was in front of me all along.

Shit! Now I have to tell him! Shit shit shit.

Within a matter of hours, we were going to be getting on separate planes – he to Iowa, me to NYC. I could not leave without telling him how I felt. I was overwhelmed with fear – what if that was not something he wanted? What if he just wanted to be friends? I thought my heart would burst at all the love that was flooding in. Oh God, how do I tell him?

As we walked toward our hotels, we held hands. That was a first. It was natural.

I said to him, "I have something I have to tell you. Can we duck into this hotel lobby for a minute?"

He said sure and then excused himself to use the men's room. I sat there thinking how am I going to say this? How how how?

He came back and sat down and those green eyes looked straight through me expectantly.

I looked back at him and said, "I'm really scared, but I think I'm in love with you."

He immediately got tears in his eyes.

He said, "I've been in love with you all this year and you never let me tell you. I had a dream six months ago where you were teaching me to fly – we sat under a tree and kissed and I sat bolt upright in bed wide awake. I was in love with you from that moment. That's why I came out to NYC, I wanted to tell you; that's why I asked you to come down and ride the elevators in Atlanta. It was my last try to tell you. Then you came with Cindy and I thought, that's it — it's not meant to be. But I didn't want to lose you as a friend."

We kissed and hugged and I sat there stunned. Oh. My. God. Things came flooding in, such as how I was just my usual self when he visited me in NYC and sometimes not very warm and friendly about his visit and he loved me anyway. *LOVED ME ANYWAY.*

All the sweet things he did for me at conferences and the letters he wrote; they were dripping with his love and I didn't see it because a part of me didn't feel I deserved it. He was too nice, and I didn't feel that kind of love was for me – I wasn't worth it.

It took me time to heal those false ideas and when they were healed, all the attraction, sexual and otherwise I should have felt before, was right there. I knew I wanted to spend the rest of my life with him.

REFLECTIONS

Instant gratification doesn't apply to real TRANFORMA-TION. Patience, discipline, visioning, consistency – those apply.

SPIRAL UP! And let everything go in their special cycles.

We have ups and downs that last for days/weeks/months/years. Perceived as "good" or"bad."

What if we just say – "I'm in a cycle?"

Menopause. A major cycle for a Queenager. It lessens. In time. Do what you can to alleviate symptoms (No advice, except fitness & nutrition!) Let your body do its thing.

Buckle up and knuckle down. Don't allow doctors to forecast your future. We love them, but ... you're in charge of your body and beliefs.

Life cycles change, as we travel to our desired level of spiritual, mental, and physical dreams.

We SPIRAL UP and the SPIRAL has rest points.

We don't jump to impossible heights on Day 1. We travel the path methodically, patiently, with intent — and keep moving.

Let go of what we think is the best outcome, and live in the moment. When we're ready, the next door will open!

A limited mindset will re-manifest the same outcomes – this was so obvious to me in my relationships with men until I met the man I married, Paul. I didn't feel I deserved to be loved in the way he was offering: unconditionally, fully, accepting me on all levels. I was living in a limiting belief system that said: YOU ARE NOT WORTHY.
When in fact, you are LIMITLESS.

It took a lot of years to understand this. Like fitness, it is not instant, not until proper cycles of awareness have been gone though. Until then, we carry a certain vibe, which changes as our thought process changes.

Your energy, vibe, frequency, thoughts are experienced as a manifested reality. How's that for WOO WOO? We are responsible for the state we're in!

Albert Einstein said:
"Future medicine will be the medicine of frequencies."

On all levels. Einstein was on to the WOO WOO. BANG BANG!

Find meditative techniques that clear your thought stream of old ideas, limiting beliefs, and clutter. Get centered with your true self; express more of her/ him/them.

SPIRAL UP & listen to cues your higher self gives you … it's real y'all.

And let your body be the outer template for the inner changes. Let it happen naturally, don't push the river, trust the process and rhythm of your special being.

TO JOURNAL

- What have you worked hard for (perhaps years) and felt the joy of accomplishment in that goal?
- What was your mindset during that time? Fixed on an outcome? A reward?
- Who supported you in accomplishing this goal?
- Fitness day-in and day-out – is a mindset. It's a way to feel that sense of accomplishment every day. Write down how the future feels, knowing you have now accomplished steps toward the goal of optimum fitness.
- How do you think, act, and approach life differently?
- After writing this down, step into this reality. You are her now! Believe it, inject it with emotion, and read it daily.

FOURTEEN

FOR THE LOVE OF DOG

I gave notice at work in NYC and by January 10th, 1989, I was driving across the country to Iowa. He had come out over the 1988 Christmas holiday to help me pack and drive a large truck of all my crap back to Iowa. I thought any man who would haul all my crap across the country must really love me!

During his visit to New York City that Christmas, we went to a party one of my boarding school friends gave. He had a cool apartment in Manhattan. He was part of the downtown crowd and his friends were all artists, photographers, designers, and very successful. Paul had not met a lot of my friends yet and my only real friend I knew at the party was the host. So we stood around and I listened to the conversations around us. I listened with some horror. There was so much talk of how much money, my book just got published, I sold a painting for $150,000, we vacationed in the south of France, blah blah blah.

He's going to think I'm like these people! I was feeling really insecure about it. Meanwhile, Paul was standing next to me eating a canape, with a contemplative look on his face.

I thought, *He's probably sorry this is going this way – he probably thinks I'm shallow like all these people at this party! He's thinking it right now!*

At that moment he looked up from his nibbling and said to me, "Wait until you taste the tomatoes in Iowa in the summer time."

The first real thing anyone had said at that party. I said, "Let's get out of here!" and we went to a movie.

I moved to Iowa and for the first time in years I had a lawn to water and a stand-alone house to live in. I had a city life for so long I forgot how other people lived. I had indeed visited Iowa before this move and found the university town to feel a little like a neighborhood in NYC. Walking around town one day, I thought, *I can do this* – (move from the big city to a small university town.) All I knew was I had to be with Paul. During that visit, I got to meet his adorable daughter, Lauren, and see where life would take us next.

We married in May, 1989. I got a design director job and we began our life together. It felt like we had always been together. The feeling of love between us created a vortex of wanting to share on a deeper level and expand this love. I could understand why lovers and life partners want to have children – something to love and nurture together and let the love grow.

I had put off ever thinking about having children. I was subconsciously not wanting to recreate a family like the one I grew up in. By the time Paul and I met, my health had deteriorated to such a point that a pregnancy could be terminal for me, the baby, or both.

But that urge to expand the circle of love became strong. Lauren, my new stepdaughter, was a wonderful addition to my life. We shared custody with her mom and she gallantly switched houses every week. She knew I loved dogs, particularly Dalmatians, and while selling Girl Scout cookies at a shopping center outside a pet shop, she told us she saw one for sale. When we went to look, it was another puppy that totally captured my heart. (In all my years of being a dog mom, I see now the terrible ways puppies are bought and sold; getting a rescue has become our method of adoption.)

This puppy was a German Shorthair Pointer – a breed I didn't know – but I was completely smitten. She was tiny, and she had a tremor – a sign from overbreeding that affected her nervous system. I didn't know that at the time. And we didn't take her home that day – Paul, as ever, needed to talk about it first. I was always one to just jump in, do it. Done.

On the car ride home, he made a case for not getting a puppy – I'd just moved to Iowa, puppies were a lot of work, we were saving our money. I loved Paul and didn't want to push him into something he didn't want to do. So, I listened, and said, "Okay." Then I feel silent as I did some inner work to let go and surrender the desire for a puppy and be okay with that. I didn't speak on the rest of the drive home as I worked on this process.

As we pulled into the driveway, Paul turned to me and said – thinking that I was brooding all the way home! – "Okay! Let's go back and get the puppy!"

We named her Tuza. She had an all-brown head with brown and white ticking in her main coat. We got familiar with the breed and decided to add to the family. That's when we got Shanti from a breeder. She also had an all brown (liver color) head, but was whiter with a roan coat. Little did we know that we now had two female alpha dogs that would spend the last eight years of their lives being separated for fear of them killing each other. I could not bear to give either one up – I was so attached to them – but we made it work by having a large house with two floors and French doors. Still, it was stressful.

Knowing I loved the breed, a co-worker invited me to come and see a new litter of German Shorthair pups a friend had. They were eight weeks old and ready for homes. *I'll just go look,* I thought. But I came home with Tobe after work – and said to Paul, "Just let him stay one night with us we'll see how it goes." Right. He never left.

He was a chill male and could sense the female alphas so he made himself fit in and was very sensitive to their moods, especially Shanti, whom he adored. His all-brown head was in stark contrast to his white coat with large brown saddle spots – and he was my heart. I had never felt this kind of connection with a pet dog before – he was just one of those special ones that capture your heart in a way nothing or no one else can. If you've had dogs, you know what I mean. If you haven't had pets, you'll think I'm crazy. He was attached to me too and would cuddle for hours – making Paul feel second fiddle. But who else would run to the door and greet me with such joy when I came home but Tobe?

Each one of our dogs has lived to be 13 or 14, even 15.

Everyone single one of them in their old age, (except for my boy, Tobe) let us know the day they were ready to cross the Rainbow Bridge.* We've had dog hospice in our home where we slept on the floor downstairs if they could no longer get up to our bedroom. Or carried them outside if they could not walk out to do their business.

When I married Paul, he and his daughter Lauren had a white fluffy cat named Costello. I never had cats growing up, only dogs. Costello was aloof and a loner. He had been passed around the sororities and fraternities in our university town and didn't really give off a feeling of permanency.

When we got our first pup, Tuza, Costello was so mad he literally pissed everywhere. I felt bad for him but he was not endearing himself to either one of us and Lauren had another cat at her mom's that was her baby. Poor Costello. I told Paul we should find him another home.

A woman and her grown son came to get Costello one day after we put the word out. I felt bad – it brought up feelings of abandonment from my own childhood but it seemed the best thing to do for Costello and to get him to a home where there were no dogs. I only hoped he had a good life.

With Tuza, Shanti, and Tobe, our house was full. There was something about Tobe that just got into my heart. He was so in love with me and would look right into my eyes when in the animal kingdom that's a challenge and not usual. But his brown soulful eyes would look into mine and I could feel this soul-to-soul connection. He was like a person, not a dog.

Other times he acted like a cat. He would weave in and out of my legs if I was washing dishes or standing in the

---

* https://www.rainbowsbridge.com/poem.htm

kitchen cooking. If I was reading the newspaper, he would come over and bat it out of my hands and give me this look – pay attention to ME! I often remarked to Paul – he's got this cat thing going on.

When he was seven, I was sitting on the couch and he was next to me. I was about to go for my daily exercise – a long walk through town. I looked at him and he looked at me. He seemed to be telling me something, but I don't know what. It was just that connection. I said "Tobe, who *are* you? And where are you going to go when you leave this furry little body?"

It was so clear to me that a soul had taken form in his dog body and that was to whom I was speaking. But something else was happening that I didn't realize until later: Tobe was saying good-bye.

The dogs had their walks earlier, so I tied my shoes and took off for my solitary stroll, thinking about Tobe and the connection we had. As I walked, I passed a church in town that had a lawn sign which always provided a witty phrase. Not a bible verse, just a clever play on words pertaining to life situations.

Today it said:
"The cat and the love you give away come back to you."

I was so shocked I went home and got my camera. I had to get a picture of this. I thought of Costello – and Tobe – nahhhh. But what if? And how? Was Tobe a reincarnated Costello? He acts like a cat.

One night Tobe hung on me and whined and cried like he never had before. It was stressing me badly. I had a hard time figuring out what he wanted. Paul and I finally got the dogs upstairs to bed next to us.

In the middle of the night, Shanti started barking, and woke us up. Tobe was having a terrible seizure. It was 3 a,m. Our small-town vet lived near us and his office was behind our house. I called Dr. Leon and told him what was going on – verging on hysteria. Tobe had come out of the seizure and was in such pain. Dr. Leon met us within 20 minutes, gave him a sedative, and checked him over.

He said, "You need to take him to the Animal Hospital at Iowa State University. I'll call them and give the referral." It was a two-hour drive in the middle of the night. We called a friend to come stay with Tuza and Shanti as we loaded Tobe into the backseat of the car – where I cradled him. He was now completely unconscious.

Hopeful and speeding, we got to the vet hospital. They took unconscious Tobe to do tests, and we waited. It was early morning, so we went for breakfast and were in the car when they called with news of Tobe's condition. Tobe had a tumor on his spine which had caused the seizure and that seizure had ruptured his brain stem. There was no hope. Paul pulled the car over and we just wept. I could not bear this news. A state trooper parked his car behind us and walked up to the driver window and asked Paul with genuine concern, "Is everything OK?"

I said, "We just got some really bad news." The trooper resembled a very close friend of ours whom we love, which brought a little bit of comfort into the moment.

We returned to the clinic where Tobe was laid out on a soft table and intubated. I asked them to take out the tube. We held him while he was euthanized. He would never animate that beautiful body again. I could not believe my boy was no longer going to be with us.

The vet administered the shot to stop his heart as I leant over and put my lips to his brown head. He took a last breath. His heart stopped. I felt a long tether was being stretched as he took his last breath and then it snapped and he was free. Gone. I could feel his gratitude to be free — but I could also feel grief beginning to crush me.

I didn't want to go home and find that Tobe wasn't there. I could hardly breathe. It was the deepest grief and pain. I closed my eyes as Paul drove us home and suddenly saw Tobe in my mind's eye. He was lying in a garden, his long front legs stretched out in front of him. He looked happy and alert – and pleased with himself. Another person – or being – was with him. This person was neither male nor female, but maybe both – and as I looked on, I realized this being loved Tobe more than I did. How was that possible!? A big yellow butterfly flitted over Tobe and the vision disappeared.

I opened my eyes and told Paul what I saw and started crying again.

I wonder if losing Tobe released the grief I had not processed from my sister's death and from the death of Louis and even facing my own death with e-coli sepsis at age 27. The grief was crushing me and it took three years to balance it out. I would be driving and think of Tobe and have to pull the car over and just weep from the depths of my being. The grief was like a heavy veil that shut out all the light. That veil had been hanging since the death of my sister, Nancy.

REFLECTIONS

The hard lessons in life have challenged my world view and my own identity. Who do I believe myself to be? Am I strong? Resilient? Capable? My early experiences gave me some confidence in these areas because I had to survive. Survival made me strong on all levels: physical, emotional, mental, and spiritual.

The big lessons have been about what we can and cannot control. We have tremendous power to guide and direct our lives in a direction that would be amazingly fulfilling and powerful, but we know it takes work and responsibility. Many people feel it's easier just to stay in one place and tread water. That's good enough.

Going in circles is a common phrase that I liken to being stuck. Going nowhere. Cycles are circles, cells are circles, the earth and planets are circles, the Flower of Life symbol, found in myriad ancient cultures with no cross-cultural opportunities to each other is made up of infinite circles. A circle is also a spiral. Like architect Frank Lloyd Wright's Guggenheim Museum in New York City, a spiral is an easy walk upwards, or downwards. Energy goes up or goes down. I like to say SPIRAL UP which means always taking it to the next level. The view is broader, the thoughts are clearer, and you avoid the downward spiral. Going in circles can be a rest point or being stuck.

TO JOURNAL

- Where are you now on your personal Spiral?
- Can you remember a time you were SPIRALING UP? What was your mindset, goals, and life like at that time?

- Have you given yourself permission to have rest points in life, or do you feel stuck?
- What parts of daily life cause stress, frustration, or sadness?
- Think of just one thing you can do to change those circumstances. Write it down.

VISION BOARD EXERCISE

- Start a vision board of what you want your life to look like.
- Put every image you can find on this vision board that expresses your BEST LIFE and look at it every day.
- Think qualities, not just material possessions.
- All you need is magazines, printed images from the internet, a glue stick, scissors and a nice big board.

FIFTEEN

YELLOW BUTTERFLIES AND DREAMS

We were walking Tuza and Shanti one early winter day on the trail bordering the plowed-under corn-fields. It was the first cold snap the previous night, trees were dropping leaves; everything was grey, including the sky. Winter was coming. We started to reminisce about Tobe, how he loved to walk that trail with Shanti – whom he adored. As we talked about him, out of nowhere, flitted a yellow butterfly like the one in my vision right after he died. A yellow butterfly on this cold winter day.

Tobe had attached himself to Shanti from day one – she was the alpha in the pack and he fell in line. He respected her so much. She would curl a lip to let him know he was crossing the line and to stop. That meant if he got up on the couch too close to her, he was greeted with a small snarl, and a lip curl. He would freeze. A minute later he would edge a little closer and she would do it again, low growl, lip curl, but allow it. He would continue this method until he was snuggled up right next to her.

She was the boss and that was fine with him.

When Tobe didn't come home with us after we had to let him go, Shanti would bark and listen for his footsteps to run down the hardwood stairs. It was clear she was calling him. When more days passed and he didn't show up, she would begin to howl and cry – she missed him so much. She would throw her head back and just howl in pain. It was heart-wrenching. Howling was something she had never done before.

One night I had a dream. I was in a big open sloping field with huge, old-growth trees dotting the hill. It was a beautiful green landscape. The sky was blocked by the size of the trees that stood like sentinels around me. I was holding a small futuristic device in my hand that told me exactly where all three of my dogs were at any given moment. I knew Tuza, Shanti, and Tobe were nearby — I could not see them, but the device showed me where they were – behind the trees up the hill, sniffing. Just then Tobe came tearing joyously down the hill toward me with Shanti chasing him happily.

I was awakened in that exact moment by Shanti who was barking, her legs moving and chirping in her sleep — something she had never done before. Paul told her to be quiet and I said, "No! She's in my dream with Tobe!"

Each time we get a dog, they bring special qualities that we need in our life at that time. Tuza brought expansive love, Shanti brought gentle peace, and Tobe brought joy and laughter. As we healed from the loss of Tobe – so unexpectedly at age 7 – about six months later I perused an ad sheet that had local puppies for sale – German Shorthair puppies. I had my heart set on one day getting another male – this one all brown with no white markings. The ad said, eight weeks, two males available, all liver (brown). Maybe I had a premonition about Kojo entering our lives.

I circled the ad and put it aside until Paul got home. *Oh hell,* I thought, and called the number. "Are the all-liver male pups still available? "

"Yes."

"Can you tell me, are they both all brown?"

"Mostly," the breeder said, "but one has some white on him."

I thought, *The all-brown one — that's ours.*

Paul got home and I wondered if it was going to be a battle about getting another dog. I gently brought the subject up. Paul looked skeptical but listened. I showed him the ad.

"Did you call them?" he asked.

"Yes."

"Do they still have them?"

"Yes."

"Then let's go," he said.

We got in the car and drove 30 minutes. After we got Tuza it was clear we were not experts at picking puppies – there were things to watch out for that impacted health and behaviors. Tuza was over-bred. Shanti was shy, which brought out aggression later to other dogs like Tuza. And Tobe, was well, Tobe.

I wanted to be sure if we got one of the liver-colored males it would be the right one for our family. At times like this I rely on getting a spiritual nudge or answer so I closed my eyes and asked God which puppy we should get. I sang that ancient word I had learned about to clear my mind of chatter and clutter – HU – and immediately the answer came: "Get the one with white on his chest."

I was disappointed. Not what I wanted to hear. *Why that one?* As I asked the question, I saw a wave of pure white light emanating from the puppy's chest that felt like pure love to me. I opened my eyes and told Paul what I had just experienced.

We got to the farm and there they were – the two male all-brown puppies – one with some small white markings. The one all-brown pup would not come near us. Very shy. His brother wanted to play with Paul's shoelaces and was happy and energetic. I knew he was the one – despite the white markings and my pre-conception of what I wanted the outcome to be.

We were thrilled to get him in the car for the car ride home. We named him Kojo – which means a boy born on Wednesday – a proper African name. I turned him over on my lap to rub his pink belly. There was a six-pointed white star on his chest – a symbol that was special to both me and Paul as it represented a high state of consciousness. It's a symbol found in ancient cultures, architecture, paintings, and photography. Think of a snowflake – or what is called the Flower of Life. We got the puppy meant for us. And he brought the love.

He managed to navigate between two cranky alpha female dogs who had little tolerance for him. He had a way of making himself very small as a presence so as not to rock the boat. His personality didn't really come out until both girls had crossed the Rainbow Bridge (died.)

Tuza went first from congestive heart failure, and Shanti about three months later. We slept downstairs with them when they could no longer get upstairs and helped them outside when they needed to go. I knew the day would come when they would let us know it was time to leave. Each one did and the vet came to our house. Both had a peaceful passing – and we knew that this was a gift we could give them – to be released from a little furry form that didn't work anymore and brought pain and suffering.

Kojo was an "only pup" for about a year and during that time we moved to San Francisco. Kojo was such a joy – so easy and well behaved. He would go to work with Paul, who was managing a commercial store. When a client would come in, Kojo would greet them at the door and take them around the place as if to show them the goods. He loved people and sometimes paid more attention to the new ones than to us.

We found Bika in San Francisco from a rescue group. The founder, Paxley, was a woman who had battled heroin and been homeless but got her life together and devoted it to rescuing dogs. She would go around the Bay Area taking dogs out of shelters, fostering them in her home and then have showings on street corners in upscale neighborhoods to find them forever families.

We were meeting friends for brunch one Sunday morning and across the street, the rescue group had volunteers talking to people, taking applications for adoptions and letting them walk the dogs around the block. We had moved to San Francisco with our beloved boy, Kojo, He was the best-behaved dog we ever had and did not skip a beat when we moved – he was just happy to come along – number four in a line of fur babies we'd had in our marriage. Tuza, Shanti, and Tobe – all German Shorthair Pointers. When we lost them one by one, Kojo was finally an only pup and his personality really came out.

As we went into the restaurant I said to Paul, "Oh, look at the dogs over there for adoption!"

He looked at me and said firmly, "We are NOT getting another dog."

We had a nice routine going with Kojo. He even had a backyard to do his business in – part of the two-story flat we rented. We were second floor, another tenant with their dogs on the first. It was an unusual property in that it did have a yard. If you did the square footage and property values in San Francisco at that time, I used to say "Kojo has a half a million-dollar yard just for him to poop and pee in." It wasn't used for anything else!

We had brunch with our friends, and then it was time to go. The rescue group was still there. I said, "Let's go over and just look!"

Paul dragged himself behind me reluctantly. There was a little orange girl pup who just looked like she wanted to be loved and nothing else. I fell for her immediately.

"Let's just walk her around the block!"

Paul didn't exactly resist, so I took her leash and they let us go around the block. She was beautiful and sweet and not so big. A cross breed of maybe Rhodesian Ridgeback and Vizsla. She had been found wandering the streets of an East Bay city alone, scared, and hungry. A local veterinarian estimated her age at nine months.

We got back to the rescue group. A table was set up and Paul walked right up to Paxley, the organizer, and said, "Can we fill out an application?"

Not getting another dog, famous last words. They had named her Eloise. A terrible name for a dog – there are no hard consonants – so we renamed her. I loved the term Habika – which means darling – and shortened it to Bika.

After the paperwork and checking us out at home, we were approved. One of the volunteers brought Bika over. Paxley said the dog shelter had told her Bika was unadoptable because she was feral. Paxley knew that was not true and took her home to foster and find her a new family. That lucky family was us.

As she came into our apartment, she saw Kojo who perked up as if to say, "Hey! A friend!" He wanted to play, but Bika was not so sure about this big brown fellow. She resisted. As the days went by Kojo started to lose interest. And he would look at us as if to say: "When is she leaving?"

Eventually they became buddies and would play tug-of-war and sleep next to each other. Bika felt safe with Kojo but she hated men with beards and pre-teen boys.

Kojo was a talker — if you petted him, he made guttural groaning noises something like a bark and a purr. He loved to be petted and scratched and would roll over on his back, loving the attention. Our flat had an east bay view — It was a San Francisco building of two floors with another flat below us. Our neighbors were a friendly gay couple, who also had a dog. Our landlord was an older couple who occasionally came to the building for maintenance.

The wife called me one day and said they wanted to buy a rug for our bedroom. There were hardwood floors everywhere but we already had a rug in our bedroom, which I told her.

The second bedroom was my art studio. The dog beds were there. Kojo and Bika would lay there while I worked, or play together. If I needed a break, I would get on the floor with them for cuddles. Kojo loved this and would let loose with his growly, guttural sounds of happiness.

So, I was confused why she wanted to get us a rug – and she said,

"Well, the boys downstairs have complained."

"About what?"

"They can hear you and your husband in your private moments."

I blurted, half laughing, "That's my dog!"

She pressed on.

"Well, we'll bring the rug over tomorrow. "

That was kind of fun. They must think Paul and I went at it all day long because Kojo was constantly moaning and groaning and I was constantly petting him when we were home.

Paul said, "Well, they're probably jealous we sound like sex addicts."

REFLECTIONS

It's so easy to make room in our lives for those things we love. Like my dogs. They fulfill my maternal instinct. Having children was not going to happen in this life due to my health. And we care for them as if they are our children. That means going wherever we go, looking after their comfort, care, health, and plenty of fresh air and exercise.

We take care of our dogs, but do we take as good care of ourselves? Do we fuss over what we are eating, getting out enough, being in the sunshine, make sure we get exercise? If you have dogs, flip the script, and see what you do for them that you are not doing for yourself.

And how about if you had children? Of course, it's the same (but way more expensive), you would do anything for them, you LOVE them. Making sure they are safe, healthy, happy, cared for.

Can you do this for yourself?

TO JOURNAL

- How can you apply the love and care you give others to yourself?
- What stops you? Feeling selfish? Not worthy? Too busy to care about self when you take care of others?
- What are three self-defeating thoughts that show up in your self-talk?
- Reframe these to encourage yourself instead and write them down.
- List one thing you can do daily for 15-20 minutes to begin self-care.

SIXTEEN

THE CHANGE AGENT

While in California we got familiar with Rhodesian Ridgebacks. They are a beautiful hound bred to chase lions off farm property in Rhodesia – now Zimbabwe — in Africa. If you look at them, they are the color of lions, have a lion-like tail and stalk like lions. If you put a wig on their head like a mane, they could be mistaken for one.

We added to our family by getting Jabu – a Rhodesian Ridgeback. Jabu is short for Jabulani which means celebration. So we had Kojo, Bika and Jabu.

Bika was immediately interested in Jabu and took over his care and education and gave him love and attention like she was his mom. Kojo had been aging fast and at almost 15 he was not interested in what those two were doing.

I was working from home, and had deadlines with freelance clients and could not attend to Jabu the puppy as much as was needed. But Bika completely took over and nannied him every day – he fell in line and adored this alpha female who was a major boss lady. This went on for months.

By now, Kojo had demonstrated behavior of brain lesions that caused him to have dementia. He was suffering and it was clear his time had come. It's never easy, but he was our fourth pup to live out his life with us and then decline to a point where the only mercy is to let them go in peace. Many people say this is so hard that they will never get a pet again. But I cannot miss out on all the love they give. With great love comes great pain in loss. But then again, love never dies, only the body form.

In 2014, after Kojo crossed the Rainbow Bridge, I found myself at a crossroads – my work life was dead and we had moved back to Iowa from San Francisco in 2009. When the economy soured, we got stuck there. The artist in me was starving for some kind of adventurous creative life, but how was I going to find it in the fields of Iowa? I had vowed never to return to the Midwest to live and here I was, age 57, stuck in the Midwest again.

As a youth growing up in Indiana, I hated the place. Everyone seemed the same – it was all white, with no diversity. If people were from a different culture or looked different from me, I wanted to know them! To be stuck again in a place without the flavor of different cultures, traditions, skin tones, ways of navigating life – I missed that.

Sitting at my computer one day I did all kinds of day-dreaming – maybe I could move to Kenya and take care of the orphaned baby elephants at the Sheldrick Foundation? Maybe there is a school in West Africa where I can teach. We had friends in Ghana, Benin, and Nigeria and we loved visiting those countries. I longed for an exotic life that was like nothing I had ever known.

I have a friend who is a change agent. She teaches people, through drawing, how to manifest what they want in their future – she provides a structure for how to go about changing your life by drawing what it is you want in your life. You don't even have to know how to draw! She's been a TED Talk speaker, authored books, and conducts international workshops for organizations and individuals to teach how to do this. She believes we are all creative geniuses and we just need to focus on what it is we want. To focus she teaches how to diagram a map and draw what it is that you want, starting from your current reality.

Because she's our dear friend, she took us through her method one day over the phone. She explained the process.

"Get a very large piece of white paper. And some colored markers."

I got a 4-foot-by-8-foot long rolled paper and taped it to our wall. We began.

"Okay. You draw your life or reality as it is now. Label it CURRENT REALITY. Then draw symbols of where you are – and no holding back: Stress? Boring? No prospects? Tight finances? Unhappy workplace? No community? You draw these things as best you can. Stick figures are fine. Whatever it is, that is your life now. Fill the left side of the page. On the right side, label it with "FUTURE REALITY." Now begin to draw symbols and things that you DO want in your life. What is the future reality you want?"

She emphasized qualities, not things, as things are transitory and qualities are what make life rich.

"Inner peace? Community? Connection? Try and keep it open since you are creating from a limited mindset at this moment and want to leave the door open for bigger things to manifest. Sure, you can put down financial abundance. That's a thing. But it's fine.

"In between these two drawings, draw three huge arrows – the three bold steps you can take right now to get to where you want your life and reality to be. Write in those arrows what those steps are."

"Quit your job, write that book, move to a new city? Whatever you can begin to do now to move toward your new desired reality. There is something about drawing these realities that releases the power for them to manifest."

Boy, did it ever.

When Paul and I put the white paper on the wall, we talked about all the things we wanted in our new reality after plumbing the current one for what was so unsatisfying. As we talked, I drew. We left this map up for months and looked at it every day. We took the three bold steps we needed to, or at least began to plan for them.

Three months later, I got an email from a university in Saudi Arabia for women. They had seen my resume online and invited me to apply for a teaching position in their fashion-design program. They were in the city of Jeddah. Jeddah? *Where's that?* I wondered. I discovered it was on the Red Sea. Oceanside living was on our map. I immediately emailed back: "Yes, I'd be very interested to apply." After interviews, they offered me the professor job.

We both got excited about the adventure, but there were so many obstacles in the way. One, our dogs. The university would provide housing for us but the compound did not accept dogs. I wanted to go so bad that I took it upon myself to call and research other compounds for expats in Jeddah that would take pet dogs. If there was no way to take our dogs, that would be a deal breaker. Either they came with us, or we didn't go.

I made calls every weekend to places I found online that housed expats. Only one took dogs and the university would pay for our housing wherever we lived. But I didn't feel they should have to find the compound that took dogs. There's not a strong pet culture in Saudi Arabia and I wanted to make sure the dogs were safe.

The one compound that took dogs, called Sharbatly, had a two-year waiting list. I asked to be put on the list. If anything at all came up, we would take it. The likelihood seemed very slim.

Meanwhile the university kept running into obstacles with hiring a 57-year-old American. The Ministry of Education said I was too old. Ha. They had rules – but in Saudi if you have "wasta," or connections, rules can be broken. The university president had wasta and found a way to get my work visa approved.

Paul and I would sit up at night in bed and talk about Saudi Arabia. How realistic was it for us to move to the Middle East with our two dogs? It didn't seem likely and the housing was a real problem.

At times I would have paralyzing fear that if anything happened while we were over there, we would not be able to get our dogs home. That was worse than not taking them.

Any change can bring up old fears, uncertainty, anxiety and the option to just shut it all down and not make any moves at all. Status quo is safe, and known. The easiest place to initialize change is with your health.

Try out new mindsets and see what this does to your day-to-day experiences. What other choices do you make? What doors open for you?

REFLECTIONS

So how does this work in changing your reality when it's your body? How long does it take?

Actually - A NANOSECOND.

Immediately.

The moment I decided to be on a path to fitness it was BANG BANG. Off and running, but not literally.
See, it happened in my mindset/thoughts/consciousness first.
IN MY IMAGINATION, WHERE TIME DOES NOT EXIST.

I held to a vision of my best self, day-in and day-out until this focused mindset and thought energy could reform the atoms that make up my body. I did this with my life overall – as I reformed what I wanted in my life – adventure and specific qualities. The Universe brought me Saudi Arabia. It fit the bill perfectly.

With fitness, I began to live the reality I wanted immediately. I visualized my ideal self inside and out. My choices aligned with this new consciousness and it was only a matter of time for the outside reality to catch up.

People ask: when did you start to see results? That might be the wrong question.

How about: When did I start to FEEL results?

That was immediate. My body began vibrating differently as I fed it nutrient-dense food and began to move my muscles. The old thoughts I'd have looking in the mirror did not exist. You know, these kinds of thoughts:

I look fat
I look old
I hate my back fat
I've got bat wings and my hind end looks huge
UGH cellulite on my thighs
Don't take my picture!

I loved my body just as it was, each step along the way.

That first step is powerful – stepping into the person you know you are and patiently doing the work to bring that into BEING. Like the sculptor Michelangelo carving the marble to reveal the Angel he saw inside the stone in his famous quote: "I saw the angel in the marble and carved until I set him free."

This is a never-ending journey of discovery – what your body can do, what your mind can achieve, and how grand it can feel to have your health and fully live your life with joy!

It's not the program/coach/diet – it's YOU.

Find the plan, make the commitment, and in the first nanosecond you will FEEL the results as you change from negative thoughts to powerful visualization of your ideal self, inside and out.

That is how to SPIRAL UP!!!

TO JOURNAL

- Write a complete description of your best self as you will be in five years. See every detail of your body, your home, your health, your style, your friends, your daily routine.
- What qualities of life do you value most?
- As our friend, the Change Agent, did with us, start making doodles and drawings of these things. You don't have to know how to draw. Just find a large piece of paper and add to it every day. Draw as much detail as you can.
- You can get her book for more details on this process:

Drawing Solutions: How Visual Goal Setting Will Change Your Life, by Patti Dobrowolski

SEVENTEEN
THE TEMPO OF TIME

The Sharbatly compound was our only hope in going to Saudi Arabia with our dogs. If they could not come, I would not accept the job. We couldn't go.

I visited the Sharbatly compound website almost every day, imagining them finding us a villa on the compound, since they took dogs. I also called other compounds, to no avail.

The Sharbatly website had a page featuring a young family – all blonds – two kids and the parents, a boy and girl around six and eight. They looked European or American and I thought for sure they were actual residents. That blond quartet became a symbol of the compound and my hopes for getting to Saudi Arabia with our dogs. Every time I went to the website this picture of the young family of four greeted me. I studied their smiles. They looked so happy. It made me feel we would also be very happy there.

The job offer came in March. It was now May and no word on housing.

We had also investigated pet transport to the Middle East. The cost was exorbitant. These companies knew they had you over an emotional barrel, and price-gouged. But we were willing to pay as so many are when it comes to your fur babies. I was to start the new job in August.

After Memorial Day, we were out running errands in the car. I checked my phone while Paul drove. An email from the Sharbatly manager, Marla. A villa had become available — a small two bedroom, did we want it?

I was so excited and immediately emailed back: Yes! We want it! It meant we could take our dogs and go!

Paul was just pulling up to the ATM drive-through of our bank. It's a small local Iowa Bank and Trust. The ATM kiosk ran ads while you waited to transact. Just after reading Marla's email and having an excited conversation, and before Paul put in the debit card, an ad showed on the kiosk. A family of four came on the screen with an ad for the bank's other services. I started screaming. Paul was alarmed until I pointed out that it was the exact same family of four that Sharbatly used on their website. What are the odds? It was a sign to me that no matter what, we were meant to go, no matter any obstacles that came our way.

When I got home, I searched image banks for "young family of four, blond" and literally millions of images were listed. How did a small Iowa bank and a compound in Saudi Arabia manage to use the same stock photo? And I thought they were real residents. Someone once said that coincidences are physical matter obeying spiritual laws.

The time quickly arrived for us to move to Saudi Arabia. I needed to go first, alone, and get permits for Paul who would be sponsored by me. He would fly a month later with the dogs. That process was incredibly stressful. We found a company in Texas that did pet transport and they fleeced us big time. They had a contact at the airport in Saudi Arabia and the forms were filled out in Arabic, but beyond that they did nothing we could not have done ourselves. But when it's your fur babies — lesson learned. Their transport was the most expensive plane ride ever taken – and it was in live cargo, not first class! We sold our car to pay for them.

I was so excited to go to this strange country I knew nothing about, have an adventure, and teach Saudi women! I read up on the customs, what to do, what not to do – but it's not really clear until you arrive.

There were major obstacles the moment I arrived.

REFLECTIONS

The tendency of life today is to be impatient. We want what we want NOW. It's hard to wait for results and if that's where our focus is, we will never be satisfied. I try to put my vision on a higher outcome and do all I can and then let it manifest. Fitness day-in and day-out. Moving to Saudi Arabia, all the steps needed to get there. Do all I can, then let go and be patient.

This is where giving up becomes very attractive. Naturally we stop doing what's not working. But what if it is working but hasn't shown up yet? There are a lot of pieces on the invisible chess board of your life and when you change your mindset, the game changes completely and pieces begin to move. Atoms rearrange. A new consciousness forms. It takes time! The Tempo of Time!

Most people give up way too early when they embark on fitness – using the bathroom scale and mirror as criteria for success only addresses the outer transformation that cannot happen sustainably without going deeper with the inner transformation. Once you KNOW you have made this nanosecond mindshift (it literally is the speed of thought!), it's like your spaceship is on course and nothing is going to disrupt your journey. I know I was meant to go to Saudi Arabia so all the obstacles meant nothing. I just kept pressing forward. It would have been easy to give up but I knew this was meant to be.

I had the same drive and knowing about my fitness journey. It was meant to be, I was locked in; it was going to fit my vision, however long it took didn't matter. In my inner being, my mindset, I was already there. I just had to be patient with the outer reality to show up and it would and it did.

TO JOURNAL

- What do you fear most? Have your fears changed throughout life?
- Write a short love letter to some object or place that makes you happy.
- What place makes you feel most peaceful? Describe that place using all five senses.
- List 10 things that inspire or motivate you.
- Write about something you knew no obstacle would stand in your way of achieving. What thoughts were in play during this time?
- How do these apply to launching a fitness journey and committing to a consistent approach?
- How can you be more accepting of the tempo of time and allow your body the time it needs to transform?
- Write down affirmations to remind yourself that your best self is already manifested and will soon appear.

EIGHTEEN

NO PLACE FOR YOU

I arrived in Saudi Arabia around 3:30 a.m. to a very large airport. The planes arrived out on the tarmac and buses picked up passengers to transport them to the main terminal. Jeddah airport is old, and it was full of men in thobes and shemagh – the long white garment of the Middle East with a red checked head scarf. The headscarves of the men were topped with a black circular agal made of goat hair to keep it in place. There were a few women, completely clad in black, faces and hands covered. You could only see a small slit in the fabric where the eyes were. Some had an additional black fabric thrown over their head and you couldn't even see the eyes. How did they see out?

I didn't have proper attire, since I had just arrived from the West. But I had deliberately worn loose, baggy clothes. I saw a man in the crowd holding a sign with my name. My driver from the university, Baksh, was waiting for me. I walked over, he greeted me kindly, and we quickly exited into the hot early-morning air. My four large bags had been lost. I was assured they would arrive the next afternoon.

It was dark, steamy, and muggy. Men were everywhere like it was the middle of the day. I found out how nocturnal Saudi Arabian society is. I had broken custom by walking into the airport without an abaya (the robe women must wear in public to cover their bodies – and I didn't have a head cover) – but it was accepted that at the airport this was going to happen when Western women arrived.

I got into the back of the van and confirmed with Baksh I was to go to the Sharbatly compound. I had no idea where I was or where we were going and I didn't know a soul where I had just landed. Baksh drove the van straddling the center line and I thought maybe this was the Saudi way of driving.

There was plenty of traffic at 4:00 a.m. Twenty minutes later we pulled off a highway, into a narrow drive lined with huge concrete barriers. This led to two uniformed guards holding assault rifles. We were at Sharbatly.
Baksh: "As salaam alaykim." (Peace be unto you.)
Guard: "Walakim Salaam." (Peace be unto you, also.)
I would get to know this greeting very well and other Arabic phrases that helped me navigate my time there.
The guard glanced at Baksh's ID and waved us through with a grimace.

We came to another security gate with an office and a drive-up window. Baksh stopped the van and the window slid open, revealing a small, brightly lit office. A large man in uniform asked our business. Baksh handed over his identification in order to enter the compound. A flurry of Arabic was spoken. It seemed there was some confusion, a problem. I put down my window and said, "I'm expected. There should be a villa ready for me." I gave my name again.

The guard shuffled some papers and looked up – "No, I don't have you on the list."

Baksh remained silent and stoic.

"Marla and I have spoken. She knows I'm arriving tonight. Here's her email."

I showed him my phone which was almost dead from the battery.

"It's villa 9-10A." It clearly said so in the email.

"Villa 9-10A?" The guard looked confused. "That one is occupied currently."

I said,

"That can't be. Marla secured a villa for me and my husband who will be arriving in a month."

The guard looked hopeful for a moment. An idea had popped in his head.

"Well, there are two women in there now, inshallah, they will let you stay with them."

My disgust and frustration began to show.

He continued, "Do you know anyone else on the compound?"

Really? I had just arrived from America and I don't know a soul in this country!

I said, "Can we just go, and see? I'm sure Marla saved it for us."

He was very doubtful and reluctant to do so. I insisted. Pushy American woman. I came to learn that you can never take no the first time. You keep at it until you get what you want.

The guard roused the compound facilities manager who had all the keys to the villas. There were 4,000 residents on the Sharbatly compound. It functioned like a small town. It was huge. It had three pool areas, a large grocery store, bowling alley, restaurants, vet clinic, spa and hair salon.

In the middle of the night all I could see was the security office and a road leading into a street lined with palm trees that had lights trained on them for effect. Every villa had a high privacy wall around it, so no dwellings were visible. Bougainvillea spilled over all the walls. It looked peaceful and tropical.

Baksh and I waited in the car with the AC on. I dozed – it took an hour. By 5:00 a.m. Maurice, the facilities manager, appeared. He was sleepy but very kind. I could tell Baksh did not want to be saddled with this newly arrived American – what was he supposed to do with me? He looked long-suffering and hopeful at the same time.

Maurice and the guard piled into a small car and we followed them to Villa 9-10 A. We stopped at a wall with bougainvillea spilling over it, and an ornate black iron gate door with colored glass for privacy. "9-10A" was painted on the stucco outer wall.

Maurice unlocked the privacy gate and we entered into a narrow, tiled courtyard. The "villa" had windows with metal shades to block out the hot Arabian sun. It resembled a fancy mobile home, but more substantial, with no front steps. It was dark.

Maurice found the key, turned the lock and I was invited to go in first. Maurice flipped on the lights in the dark villa. I half expected a couple of screaming women to emerge in their pajamas. No one was living here. It was stifling.

It had clearly been set up to receive new residents. There were packages of new bedsheets and pillows from IKEA on the bed. It had been recently cleaned. The guard went to each room and put the AC on full blast and then these three men stood back with bated breath to see my reaction.

I was so tired.

I said, "Okay, I guess this is it. It's fine."

It was small but it looked clean and here I was finally in Jeddah, Saudi Arabia! There was visible relief on everyone's face and the guard became quite jovial at that point.

"We are happy you are here! Marhaba! Welcome to Sharbatly!"

I had other concerns.

"Where is the office so I can see Marla in the morning?"

I knew nothing about what was where on the compound.

The guard said kindly, "Oh don't worry we will come and get you in the morning, inshallah. We will bring you to Marla, inshallah. What time would you like us to come and get you? 11?"

It was 5:30 am now and I was exhausted.

"Thank you, but can you come at 12:30 instead?" I needed to sleep.

"Okay! We will come and get you at noon, inshallah! Good night!"

The three of them left and I unpacked the new bed linens and made the bed. I had no clothes, no baggage, and there was nothing to eat or drink. No toilet paper. At least it was clean and quiet!

And I was absolutely thrilled to be in Saudi Arabia! My dream of adventure, exotic location, different culture, a life with qualities I longed for was just beginning.

REFLECTIONS

The superpower we all have to use our thought and intention to manifest a life we long for, with qualities we desire to experience, is ready and waiting for us. It takes mindset work to put this into play. Too often we waste thought energy on worry, negative thinking, pessimism, or news bingeing, and information overload. Our superpower requires FOCUS.

Choose what you think – the thought is like a river, a stream in which we throw all kinds of polluted junk. We then wonder why our life is full of polluted junk – what we read, eat, think about, accept each day – fills our thought stream and our bodies. Is it time to declutter? Pivot completely? CLEAN OUT and SPIRAL UP?

Gratitude is a "clean river thought." It sparkles. It cleans up the crap we've thrown in our thought stream.

Take care of this magnificent chariot for the Soul through high-quality nutrition and structured exercise. You can do it. Your body wants to be strong and healthy!

TO JOURNAL

- What daily habits can you change that will help put you in a positive frame of mind? (For example, looking at your vision board.)
- Write down three things you are grateful for every night before going to sleep.

- Try "fasting" from reading news, watching TV, being on social media for one day or a half-day a week. What does that feel like?
- What are your core values? Are you living your life in accordance with them?
- List 10 things that inspire and motivate you.

NINETEEN
CAGED MONSTERS

I woke up at 1:30 the next afternoon. No one had come to my door. No one had come to get me! So, I poked my head out the door of my villa and walked to the privacy gate. I opened the gate and stuck my head out. I saw the bright Arabian sun and felt the hot day and thought *Where am I, really?*

I was in a huge compound in a strange country and I had no idea where I was or how to get to anyone who knew. No one was around. Just gated walls, private invisible villas, and feral cats everywhere. The cats sat on the walls, prowled the street and were in such abundance I wondered who fed them all. Some were huge tom cats and looked ferocious. Groups of cats clustered with the same color and markings. *Kittens must be born every day,* I thought.

I closed the gate and wondered what to do. I considered crying. I thought if I was the type of woman who cried in the face of impossible obstacles, now would be a good time. But I'm not. So instead, I went outside again and saw a car approaching. I waved him down. A nice man from Lebanon allowed me to get in his car and dropped me at the compound rental office. It would have been a good 20-minute walk in the hot sun without me knowing where I was going.

Marla, the rental office manager, was all smiles. She was South African and made me an espresso. She had messed up big time but didn't mention it. Neither did I. She took me to the compound store to get water, toilet paper, and some food. She drove me back to my villa after showing me the directions of the pools, spa, and restaurants. It was a hasty tour accomplished by waving her arms. Still, it took me a week to find anything – I had to stop and ask any resident I saw walking about.

When I got back to my villa it was just about prayer time. In a few moments it began. There was a mosque on practically every corner in Jeddah, and one on the compound. The haunting quarter tones of the muezzin captivated me. I stuck my head outside the door to hear better, lifted my face to the sun, and closed my eyes to listen to the ancient call to prayer. I was in Saudi Arabia and I already loved it.

Many people who move to Saudi Arabia report the miracles that happened to get them there. It was as if certain souls were meant to be there for specific unknown purposes beyond the job they were hired to do.

I knew with the "family of four" picture coincidence that whatever obstacle arose in our move to this country, it was meant to be – and it would happen.

A month later, our dogs were put on a flight out of Chicago, and Paul followed on another close behind. As usual, planes arrived in Saudi Arabia in the middle of the night due to the excessive heat. I had some new friends drive me to the airport to get Paul. They were a young couple from Germany and knew how things worked and how to help someone out. That was the thing – it was so easy to meet new friends in Saudi Arabia, from all over the world.

The Jeddah airport became one of my favorite places to move in and out of, not because it was in any way luxurious, as it wasn't – it was more a third-world airport, like the ones I had experienced going in and out of West Africa. I loved it for the same reasons I loved the African airports — there was such a wave of humanity that came through from all over the world. And in Jeddah, Muslims were on their sacred pilgrimage to Mecca, which was only 40 miles away up in the Hijaz Mountains, east of the Red Sea.

I loved the humanity I saw in the airport, with small brown withered women wrapped in colorful fabrics from India, giving me a toothless grin. Or the families of people coming to experience Haj – the holy pilgrimage to Mecca – looking like matching dolls. The people from Pakistan, India, Kuwait, Oman, Syria, Egypt, Africa, Indonesia – sometimes in big groups together – where they all wore matching hijab and had the name of the tour company printed on their backs.

I loved witnessing these spirits in form – so many different cultures, languages expressing life through their bodies, and felt the ultimate observer of God's grace seeing these souls come through the airport – often with nothing more than a wrapped bag of belongings, clutching a passport.

The Saudi men at the check points for customs were professional, friendly, and beautifully groomed in their white starched thobes and red checked shemagh head scarf. When they saw I was a resident they always said "Welcome home!"

Even though I would never be able to call it my permanent home.

Paul arrived at 3:00 a.m. He was not hard to pick out of a crowd in the arrival area. Tall, slim, white, and American in a sea of Arabs who tended to be short, dark, and portly. It was such a happy reunion! Here he was with me in Saudi Arabia! We had decided he would retire, since I was the reason we were here, hired to work as a professor at an all women university, Dar Al Hekma.

It was several hours before we could pick up the pups. They arrived later and we had to hire a van to get them. They had been taken to the cargo hangar and the paperwork was taped all over their kennels with their names written in Arabic (I had taken lessons before leaving for Saudi). I was so stressed waiting to see my babies to make sure they were okay.

We got to the cargo hangar. They were brought out on a front loader, both panting and stressed. I ran over to them and was admonished by a stern man to wait until they were put on the ground. Somehow, we got them in the hired van, all the while I could not let them out of their transport kennels. There were a few French fries in each kennel. It was clear someone had tried to feed them. Though they had water and food, it was still a 24-hour ordeal that had a pit-stop in Frankfurt, Germany where vet techs checked on live cargo. We didn't know if there had been enough time for them to have been checked.

Once back at our new home – Villa 9-10A, they were let out, happy, but exhausted.

Dogs were pets in Saudi Arabia, mostly owned by royalty as guard dogs. People didn't understand pet culture and would get a puppy for their small child, not know how to train the pup, and as it got older, discard the dog on the street. There were many organizations that picked up abandoned dogs and found them good homes. German Shepherds were commonly abandoned and rescued, as well as all other breeds. An Australian friend ran a rescue group for abandoned dogs and would arrange for adoptions abroad – in the U.S. and Europe.

There are strict laws about dogs coming in and out of Saudi Arabia and some breeds are not allowed: Chows, Rottweilers, and Pit Bulls, for instance. Many of the German Shepherds that were abandoned and then rescued by my Aussie friend were adopted in the U.S. and became K-9 Dogs with a police force. It was so heart-warming to see them given a new life.

We had friends from South Africa that had two Chows when the husband was offered a great job with Pepsi — in Jeddah. They were one of the really wonderful expat couples we met in Saudi Arabia. Chows Zita and Zorro were not breeds allowed in Saudi Arabia. Paperwork for dogs being brought in had to be strictly followed – and at the top was the name of the breed.

Our friends knew they would never get in with their Chows. Like us, leaving them behind was unthinkable. So, they asked their vet to change the breed to "Labrador Retrievers." Any dog that was a guard dog or a hunting dog qualified to come into Saudi Arabia, except the ones mentioned. Even a small yippy Yorkie was welcome. After all, they are guard dogs, announcing intruders.

When Zita and Zorro arrived from South Africa the customs people – who didn't know a Chow from a Chihuahua, waved them through without a hassle.

I learned that the best way to get through customs was to smile, say a few Arabic words and express my joy at being back in Jeddah. It was genuine joy, and was amazing how it worked. We traveled once outside the country, taking Jabu with us. We were living in Florence for the summer. Jabu's kennel did not go to the cargo hangar but arrived by coming up the baggage conveyor belt ready to slide down to the carousel. It caused a huge scene, but Paul was able to get two baggage handlers help get the kennel off the belt before it hit the bottom.

Poor Jabu!

I took him to the customs area, his kennel on a huge flat cart. I knew enough Arabic to make jokes about the monster dog in the cage. The supervisor came out looking very stern, but then broke into a smile when I spoke Arabic. Everyone wanted to see the exotic animal in the cage. They waved me through without even looking at the paperwork. They were distracted by an American woman, speaking Arabic with a caged monster in tow.

The compound we lived on had a gym open 24 hours. It was well equipped and well used due to the heat. The pool was an option for non exercisers. Despite being mostly covered up in public in Saudi Arabia, on the compound you lived a Western lifestyle. Pool, bathing suit, no gender segregation. My job was extremely enjoyable, low stress, and fulfilling. I was again determined to use this time to get fit. I started a new program, another restrictive way to eat – with specific foods on specific days. It was exhausting and not worth all the work it took to lose 8 pounds over 2 months. I gave up but kept going to the gym despite now putting those 8 back on. I had maybe one good week at the pool feeling confident in my body.

REFLECTIONS

I've learned that Fitness is a body, mind, spirit endeavor – addressing all three WHEELS OF SELF will bring lasting success and stupendous TRANSFORMATION. Your friends and family will see a trimmer, healthier you, but inside that chariot for your Soul is the landscape of real dreams alive and well.

I had fitness of mind and spirit at this point in my life, but not of the body.

Fitness is also how you feel, think, and BE. It all comes to a fine arrowpoint in your body that will show the hard inner work you have done and manifested out here.

It's the only thing worth pursuing – inside – a self-love and self-awareness that leads to living a life of your dreams.

By the way, whatever I write is stuff you already know yourself. I am just reminding you. That's why it resonates.

You are already the Strong, Fit, Queenaging, Bad Mamma Jamma, Brick House of Beauty that lives in your dreams. She's you. Let her out. C'mon!

We have navigated life this far with such success and it's time to start a revolution of showing the world just how fierce women in their 50's, 60's, 70's and 80's can be. However that looks to you! Just BE YOU! BE!

You are a human being not a human doing. A magnificent BEING that's you.

Don't just DO YOU, BE YOU!!!

SPIRAL UP!

TO JOURNAL

- What part of you is that Strong, Fit, Queenaging, Bad Mamma Jamma , Brick House of Beauty?
- Who has seen her?
- How can you bring her out again?
- What does she feel like?
- Complete this sentence and then keep writing: "I am courageous because I _____."

TWENTY

THE LITTLE GENTLEMEN

In general Saudis loved Americans and treated us well. After that came the Brits, then Germans, then South Africans – at the bottom were Filipinos and Pakistanis and Indians. Sadly, racism exists everywhere. Having brown skin was not a factor in racism. There are all skin tones in Saudi Arabia. Many Africans settled there in the early part of the 1900's and were invited by the first king, Al Saud, to become permanent, passport-holding Saudis.

After a year at Sharbatly, we wanted to move out. The place eventually felt small and frankly my American compatriots were a drag to be around. While I was loving being there, so many complained about the country – the people and the conditions. They were there for the money only – and brought their American life with them and all those expectations and prejudices, and laid them over their new life in Saudi Arabia. For them, Saudi Arabia simply did not fit. Complaining was the topic of any conversation with most other Americans. They assumed you felt the same. I did not feel the same. Neither did Paul.

Paul got a mountain bike and found a tribe of guys from all over the world with which to ride up in the desert mountains. It became his great joy. Because most of them worked, they would get up at 4 a.m. and ride for a couple of hours until sunrise. The mornings were cooler. The weekends were longer.

As they rode to the outskirts around Jeddah, where there were no houses, they would come upon Bedouins in tents who were delighted to see them. They'd offer tea, and want to talk even though there was no English on their part and no Arabic on the cyclists' part. But it was a connection that both sides enjoyed, and it happened often.

I have a picture of Paul riding in the desert looking like a Tour de France athlete in his bicycling outfit, riding past a Bedouin on a camel, holding a cell phone. The Bedouin is looking at Paul, like WTH? and also speaking into the phone. I wish I knew what he was saying in that moment he passed Paul. They shared a look. Paul waved and moved on.

We moved out of the compound. I had to sign a paper with the university saying I took full responsibility for my own safety. I did that anyway! The U.S. government wanted U.S. citizens on guarded compounds – but I found it suffocating and negative.

To be clear, I never felt safer in my life than when we lived in Saudi Arabia. The government (Royal Saudi family and appointed ministries) keep a tight rein on the people. Breaking laws had swift and dire consequences. The populace mostly behaved admirably but there were pockets of criminal activity in the eastern provinces. Any laws that were being broken, like drinking alcohol or transporting and taking drugs, were happening with the younger royal family members, which numbered into the thousands. There is always a way around rules when you are in the power seat and have "wasta."

Our new villa was in an unguarded compound and we lived among Saudis, Egyptians, Syrians, Lebanese, Africans, and others. One of my colleagues was a department chair from Finland and we enjoyed a close friendship with her and her husband.

The dogs were welcome at this compound and once we moved in, there would be knocks at the door all day and night from the kids on the compound wanting to see the dogs – of whom most were terrified.

I had a driver that took me to and from school. His name was Elias – he was the brother of Baksh – and his English was terrible, so he spoke in a combination of guttural grunts, Urdu, and Arabic. He was originally from Pakistan but had lived in Saudi Arabia his entire life. He had children and one day he somehow managed to express that he wanted to bring his 7-year old son in the car so he could meet my dogs. His son had never seen a dog up close before.

Each time Elias came to pick me up in the morning, Paul would walk me to the privacy gate of our villa in Sharbatly and Bika and Jabu would poke their heads out and they'd all say good-bye for the day. So Elias knew we had dogs.

One time Elias said to me, "Mr. Paul – Hulk Hogan. Same same."

I laughed. Hardly, but okay. Elias enjoyed seeing Paul when I was dropped off or picked up and Paul made a point to come out and say hello, both in the morning and evening. I didn't always have Elias as my driver, they switched up every month. There was Muhammed from Eritrea who honked and winked at the African maids on the compound every time he drove through, and the very quiet and stoic driver M – whose wife had cancer and at the university we all gave donations for her care. The drivers did not make much money.

Baksh dropped me off at home one time and I realized I'd forgotten my phone in his car. I used Paul's phone to call him and he drove back – 30 minutes each way – an extra hour in total to get my phone back to me asap. I was so appreciative I gave him a huge tip of 100 riyal – about $25 U.S. I knew that Baksh had two wives and five children.

Elias managed to ask me about bringing Abdullah, his 7-year-old son, on the ride home. to see my dogs. I texted Paul to be prepared - we had a visitor coming. I told him the scenario and to get the dogs ready. When we arrived, Elias and his son got out of the car and Elias pushed his son toward the dogs. Abdullah screamed. He was scared of them. Elias grabbed his hand to pull him closer and Abdullah resisted and started to cry. This sweet boy who had just been helping me count in Arabic in the car.

I intervened and told Elias, "It's okay. Let him go."

I stooped down and invited Abdullah to touch the back of Jabu – our most mellow dog. Elias hesitantly came over and I took his hand and slowly and gently rubbed it over the ridge on Jabu's back. Jabu stood there patiently, not moving. I was practically moved to tears seeing the joy on Abdullah's face when I realized this was the first time he had ever touched or been close to a dog.

Wherver we went, and with all the friends we had that were Saudi, it was the little boys who loved the dogs most and wanted to touch them. I have so many pictures of the little gentlemen of Saudi Arabia tenderly petting Jabu and Bika.

REFLECTIONS

Fear and joy can live side by side. We decide which side we want to be on. Sometimes we just need someone to show us. With fitness and getting our bodies back to where we want them in health, strength, and size after years of neglect, we've built up a wall of indifference. As we approach this wall it brings up fear.

We have no idea how to get what we want. It's all too overwhelming unless someone shows us how it's done. If you can afford it, it's worth getting a personal trainer, but more valuable is getting over your fears. Fears of going to the gym and looking silly or like you don't belong, fears of being on a deprived, restrictive diet, fears of failure.

But if you overcome your fears, it will bring joy like you have not experienced in a long time. Those first times you see muscles develop, and your clothes fit looser, your eyes sparkle with health and you feel amazing.

It takes time, unlike the time it took Abdullah to go from fear of dogs to the joy of a new experience petting one – but you can do it.

TO JOURNAL

- What fears do you have around fitness? Write each one down.
- Under each fear write down three things you can do to face that fear or change your mindset from fear to curiosity.
- Take one step tomorrow on one thing you wrote down to face a fear.
- At the end of the day write how it felt, what helped or hindered you, what you can do tomorrow.

TWENTY-ONE

STRONG WOMEN

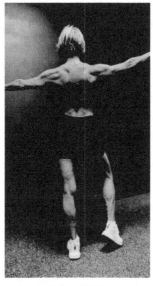

Julia, 2022

S ome of the dear women I met in Saudi Arabia had stories that we in the West do not understand. I met a dear friend, Noor (not her real name). She was my age who had grown up in Indonesia in a wealthy family. The grandfather was the patriarch, and more than the father he called the shots. They were Muslims.

When Noor turned 12 and her period started, her grandfather took her out of school and married her off to one of his friends – an old man. Noor had a baby at 13 and the marriage turned out to be a disaster, as he was unkind and abusive. So Noor was allowed to leave that marriage and return to school. She now had a son whom her family took care of. She returned to school for an education – and she was very smart.

When she was 17, she went on a school trip to Florida. There she met a young man from Saudi Arabia who was studying at the university. They fell in love quickly and he invited her to come and live with his mother and father in Jeddah while he finished school. She moved to Jeddah and was warmly accepted into the family, and they were married.

She raised a family, and had also created numerous businesses that benefitted women. She hired Filipino women in her businesses – and she treated them very well, which is usually not the case. They were given a salary, clean accommodations, transportation to and from work, time off to go home, plane tickets paid for.

Noor and I often talked about the mysteries of life. There was so much gratitude and life in this woman – who was my age and had such a different upbringing and life experience. We felt like sisters and she had a rebellious streak I loved. She was a chic woman of the world who I met at a fashion event, and we were immediately drawn to one another.

Women were banned from driving in Saudi Arabia until 2018. But Noor would dress up like a man with a shemagh and white thobe and take the car for a spin around Jeddah. Women had been put in prison for such antics – but Noor remembered when Jeddah had nightclubs and women were not required to cover up.

An attack on Mecca in 1979 caused the Saudi ruling family to make a deal with the conservative religious imams in order to stay in power. Women would now be required to cover and could not drive. Other laws were put in place that stole women's freedom, but after a generation it became the norm.

After King Abdullah died in 2016, King Salman, a half-brother, took power after a decision by a group of elder princes. It was said the King appoints a crown prince (second in line) as well. King Salman was the new king and Prince Muqrin, another half-brother, was the crown prince.

Saudi Arabia had a line of princes become Kings in their old age and some did not last very long. Muqrin was older – late 70's. Maybe it was because of this that the crown prince designee was changed to Prince Nayef, a favorite of the U.S. government for his collaborative work on the war on terror. He had close ties to Washington.

Then suddenly, Prince Nayef was out – placed under house arrest — and Prince Mohammed bin Salman was named Crown Prince. He was a son of King Salman, but brash and young and had not been educated abroad. King Abdullah had at one time banished him from the palace – he had displeased the King for something. His age was around 35, it was said.

He is called MBS for short. He wanted to modernize Saudi Arabia and lifted the ban on women driving but also imprisoned women who had defied the ban before it was lifted – as if to say it's not because of your activism that this is happening, but due to my largess.

Despite the politics of Saudi Arabia, we felt removed from the drama. My colleagues and new Saudi friends were not so removed, as many of them had family fortunes threatened if someone displeased MBS.

News was censored and I have to say it was a relief. Also, a relief was the lack of marketing and bombardment of holiday decorations and buying frenzies especially around Christmas. Many had a hard time giving that up, but not me – it was a relief. My memories of family Christmases were not happy, nor were Paul's, so after Lauren went to college, we stopped the whole tradition and concentrated on just being with friends and family over a great dinner. Maybe some Christmas lights outside; that was it. No tree, no spending money on things we didn't need or want.

REFLECTIONS

Women supporting other women is a powerful intentional force. A fitness journey is a golden opportunity to find your sisters in health, walk the path together, support each other, celebrate wins, and find the strength when you need it. Collective wisdom in a group of women Queenagers is off the charts. Remember how wise our grandmothers were? They had lived some life! Now you have too, and you are wise beyond what you know.

Fitness communities are powerful tools for transformation. We don't do this alone, it's very hard to sustain alone. But when you are on a team of a group of women dedicated to the same goals, it's life changing.

Sometimes getting fit and healthy is threatening to friends and family. You might have to move into new circles of friends who support your goals and understand its importance to you.

As you change your life style and daily habits, it can disrupt relationships in subtle ways. Transformation is on many levels and if you feel shattered about any of it, just know the pieces will come together again and fit better than they did before.

You deserve to be happy, healthy and free of negativity from inside yourself, or outside.

TO JOURNAL

- Pick one thing that's standing in the way of your dreams. What could you achieve if that one thing was removed from your life?
- Who do you trust most? Why?
- What are your strengths in relationships (kindness, empathy, etc.)?
- How do you draw strength from loved ones?
- What do you value most in relationships (trust, respect, sense of humor, etc.)?

TWENTY-TWO
IT JUST LOOKS DIFFERENT

In Saudi Arabia, I was exposed to the idea of multiple wives and learned the different ways this happened. One young lady I worked with, Lina, (not her real name) who was 26, told me about her family one day. She had never met an American and I adored her sweetness and openness and we had many conversations. She was one of three children. Her parents married when her father was 15 and her mother 14. It was arranged. They had the three children and all of them were now in their 20s, still living at home, which is the tradition until they marry and get their own homes. Lina told me her father came to her mother a few years ago, and asked if she was okay if he took a second wife. She said, if it will make you happy. Just don't bring her to Jeddah.

Lina explained that her parents loved each other but were not long IN love with each other. It's common for a man to move on from his first wife, but not divorce her and throw her out. She remains an important member of the family with a level of respect. And she is cared for financially, still considered an important family member, mother of the first-born children. She has a separate house from another wife (or wives.) It must be equally resplendent in all ways as the other wife's house.

The second wife came into being and Lina's father had a daughter with her. As Lina's mother got used to the new arrangement, the second wife moved to Jeddah and now the family, as one, spend time together. Who can say how the women were feeling about this? From the outside a woman who is no longer in love with her husband nor he with her, is not relegated to poverty as an outcast. Many would have no place to go.

Another situation was my friend Lujain (not her real name.) She is from Pakistan, had married young to a man she thought she loved. But as the years went by and they were unable to conceive, it bothered him greatly. She was also an independent woman from a wealthier family. Her marriage was not arranged – she chose him. They decided to adopt, since a baby was not forthcoming and they wanted children. Her mother, knowing this, got a call from a female doctor friend who was working in Pakistan at a refugee camp full of people fleeing Al Qaeda. The doctor called Lujain's mother and reported, "I have a baby for Lujain if she is ready to receive her."

A young woman of 16 came into the camp with her parents, in a very late-term pregnant state. She gave birth to the baby, but promptly died. The parents left the camp without the baby and never returned. The doctor told Lujain's mother, "This baby will die tonight if no one takes her and cares for her." Lujain agreed as did her husband and a nurse drove through the night in a taxi to deliver the newborn to Lujain and her husband.

Things did not go well with the husband, and Lujain eventually divorced him. When the adopted daughter was a few years old, suitors arrived looking to marry Lujain, an educated women from a wealthy family – but more often than not they would ask her to give the girl back to where she got her – they didn't want someone else's child to raise. Especially a refugee camp child whose lineage was unknown. Lujain was incensed and would say, "She's not some pet I can return!" She was outraged by the men who suggested this.

Eventually a man approached her who was high up in the government. As he got to know her, he was very touched that she had adopted this child from a refugee camp and that the baby would have died that night if Lujain had not accepted her. He said he wanted a wife with that kind of heart and asked her to marry him. Lujain said yes.

He had his own story to tell. He had two children himself. His wife had been in an accident many years before when the children were toddlers. She had a brain injury that reduced her to a vegetable state. He couldn't bear to put her in a home, so he took care of her at home and hired nursing care. He never divorced her. So Lujain became his second wife and to this day she helps care for the first wife with loving care and has accepted their children as her own.

When you hear of second or multiple marriages, it's foreign to Western sensibilities but in other parts of the world where harsher realities exist and other traditions have been followed, it is not what it seems.

I had a Saudi woman colleague in her forties who was considering becoming the second wife of a wealthy Saudi. She talked it over with me and said,
"Financially I would be taken care of and be able to travel with him but not have to sleep with him every night!"

It seemed the perfect solution for a woman who had been married once, and was a single mother. She was excited about the possibility. It made sense even to my Western perspective.

Another experience that was jarring and a frequent occurrence in Saudi was capital punishment. Before we got our own car, we hired drivers to take us places – when we wanted to eat out or go to the beach. There were special beaches for expats, bikinis and all. Early on, a few became our regular drivers. One of them was so happy to give us a tour of Jeddah the first few months we arrived. Tahir was from Pakistan and delighted in showing this American couple all the sights around Jeddah like the huge art sculptures on the Corniche (coastal drive), prince's palaces, and government buildings. I would be snapping photos from the backseat.

Tahir pulled into a parking lot and pointed to a sign that had a camera with a red slash through it. "No pictures," he said in his sing-song, jovial voice. I saw a white canopy over a raised platform that had white tile on the surface. It was the size of a two-car garage.

As we rounded the structure Tahir said in a happy voice, "This be where they are chopping heads after noon prayer on Fridays. See, there is the Ministry of the Interior across the street."

People would crowd the platform to witness this on Fridays. An executioner skilled in using the sword was employed to do the job. We heard from other male expats that some had gone to witness such a horrible event (who knows why!) and being a foreigner, were pushed to the front for a better view. God forbid.

REFLECTIONS

One huge benefit of living abroad is in accepting others within the culture in which they live and realizing that beneath it all, we are all the same. We are humans on planet earth doing the best we can to live the life we have.

It used to take generations for attitudes to change in a society, now it takes a few years, sometimes just months, as new ways of thinking spread through communities. The fitness model for women, for instance in the 1980's was aerobics. Actress Jane Fonda created the first aerobic workout tapes in 1982, with leg warmers, step aerobics, and tights.

There is no such thing as getting "toned." Your muscles either shrink or grow, get hard or stay soft. "Getting toned" was a marketing term to appeal to women. Luckily this has changed in a few decades, but lifting weights will not make you bulky or look like a man.

The women bodybuilders who do get bulky and huge want to look that way, and take certain performance-enhancing drugs to get that way. Unless you do too, you aren't going to get bulky.

We think we have an understanding of something when really it simply doesn't fit our thinking, because it looks different.

If we are prone to judge others, it most likely is also our weak spot – we judge ourselves. What bothers us most in others is a reflection of us, mirrored back to us, as annoyance or outright hatred of someone. It's the old saying: "You spot it, you got it."

TO JOURNAL

- What qualities do you see in others that set you off or cause annoyance? When do you engage in the same behaviors?
- How do you secretly feel about someone who is obese?
- Do you have any of the same feelings about yourself (even if you are not obese, but maybe overweight?)
- How do you secretly feel about someone who is slim and healthy?

TWENTY-THREE

THE SISTERS AND THE VILLAGE GRANDMOTHER

The all-women university where I taught fashion design organized trips every few months – sometimes to another country or other parts of Saudi Arabia.

There was an architectural conference planned by the university to go to Asir, a province in the south of Saudi Arabia near the Yemen border. We were going to partner with leaders from the area to implement a plan to preserve the Arabian stone dwellings and historic buildings in that area. Many of the archeological sites in Saudi are not being actively investigated. There has been resistance to anything that predates the appearance of Prophet Mohammed 1,400 years ago and the beginning of Islam.

This village was up in the mountains of Asir. We took buses full of our students to the site and decamped at a local hotel. There were three days of talks and presentations, and the small village that hosted us also created a kind of festival of local arts and crafts.

This was an extremely conservative area and we were advised not to wear anything colorful – such as our abayas and head scarves. Everything should be black. As faculty, we didn't have to cover our faces, but many of the students did.

We arrived at the village. There was a large, central outdoor area surrounded by stone dwellings. Shocking pink banquet chairs were set in front of a makeshift stage, under the open sky. The bright pink chairs were a contrast against all the black being worn by the women.

Between presentations, I sat with my sketchbook and drew. A few women who spoke good English asked if I would come sit with them. Of course! They had probably never met an American. They asked me to draw them – which I did, as I found out that four of them were sisters and one was a family friend. They pointed out their mother sitting at a table selling food and she brought over a plate for me.

I drew each young woman, concentrating on there beautiful eyes. Even with heads and faces fully covered, I could find the individuality of each face. I underscored this by writing their names below the portraits done with marker on paper.

The warmth and genuine feeling of hospitality is something Arabs are famous for and they were not an exception. Later in the day as I continued to sit with them, I drew all four sisters, their friend, their two little brothers, the mother and numerous other children who came up and wanted to be drawn. Traditional music was being performed and one of the sisters stood and invited me to follow her movements. She showed me their traditional dance and we linked arms. She showed me how to face front and kick my feet forward gently. We were having a grand time when an old man – clearly very conservative — gave us the evil eye and motioned for us to stop. My dancing partner didn't react or flinch; she just laughed and sat down.

Later I was with my colleague from Finland. We were invited to have some tea, handed to us graciously by a woman fully covered in black. We could only see her warm brown eyes, crinkling at the corners. She invited us into her home which was up some stairs of a very old stone dwelling. Traditional floor and back pillows lined the walls of the room. She took off her hijab, revealing an incredibly gorgeous face of about 35 years of age.

Later we went back downstairs and were met by a young man who wanted to give us a tour of the art exhibit that had been set up for the occasion. As we were shown the work, a boy of about eight tagged along. There were other boys in the village that age, but they were wild and running about with abandon — not very well behaved. They were normal kids in play clothes, looking like ragamuffins. But this boy was self-contained, with a noble sense about him, a strong presence, like a little man. He was impeccably dressed in the tradition of Saudi Arabia. A starched, bright white thobe and red checked head wrap. His dark brown eyes were sparkling and happy. I thought: *This boy is so loved.*

The tour guide, a man of about 25, seemed like an older brother to him. But he explained to us that the boy was an orphan and that the whole village looked after him. The main person who looked after him was a woman they called "grandmother" and he invited us to meet her. We said good-bye to the eight-year-old little man and my Finnish friend and I were led to a house in the small village. We entered and a very small, brown, wrinkled woman – ageless but definitely old – how old I have no idea – maybe 80 or 90 — was there completely covered as in the Saudi tradition. He introduced us in Arabic and she nodded her head to us. He said she is the one who cares for all the orphans in the village including the boy you met. Then he left us with her. Here was the Queenager of Queenagers – her small stature, but noble posture, exuded gentle energy and a strong presence. She removed her face covering to reveal a gentle brown face. The beautiful Grandmother of Orphans.

I leaned over and kissed this little withered woman on the forehead which was the tradition in Saudi Arabia with elders to show respect. My Finnish friend and I dug in our purses for riyals to donate to her for the care of the orphans. She gave a nod with a toothless grin and disappeared. Of all the women I met in Saudi Arabia, she held the energy of a kind of Love Goddess, one who dispenses love to all the children who are without parents in her village and takes care of them. The impeccable nature of the young boy we met proved how well she does her job.

Later that night we had a huge feast. The village leaders had arranged for goats to be roasted and vats of Saudi honey and dates, vegetable dishes, Arabic bread, hot tea and other goodies to be served. I had noted with sadness that all the bleating sounds of the goats from earlier in the day had now ceased.

Men sat at one end of a very long makeshift table and women on the other, not across from each other. We sat on cushions on the ground. There must have been 80 people seated, men and women, segregated.

The next morning came a warning. Some of the more conservative men of the village objected to our female students wandering the paths of the village in the dark, even though there were spotlights set up here and there. They had witnessed groups of young men talking to young women which set off alarm bells and they reported this to the local Ministry of the Interior. One man drove all night to Jeddah to report it to the proper officials.

Our university leader, including our provost and president — both Saudis with doctorates — shrank at the suggestion of impropriety and suggested no one go back to the village the next day. The female students were not welcome. It was a shock and disappointment but typical for how fast things can change in Saudi Arabia! The provost was from this area of Asir – and should have known what line could not be crossed.

Saudis are some of the most tech-savvy people in the world. Everyone owns a phone. Congregating in either mixed company or as a group can threaten the ruling family, so people use texting and communicating on phones and social media. That is also closely watched.

The sisters I drew, and their mother, all had Instagram accounts and we shared those with each other before our departure. We have remained in contact, which is such a blessing to me.

One of the famous village sons was a fashion designer who left as a young man and went into the fashion business creating haute couture garments for wealthy clients. His claim to fame was a dress he designed for Princess Diana – when she was with Dodi Fayed, the Saudi who died with her in in the car accident in Paris. That dress was on display in the village as a testament to the talent that came from that region. Later I met the fashion designer and knew him already from his connection to my department chair. He kindly helped me negotiate a fair price for a textile piece, a traditional craft that came with five different stories of who made it.

In some ways, Saudi Arabia is a small country It's so tribal and news travels so fast. People seem to be connected at a certain level of socio-economic status. They all know each other despite distances – just by the family names.

Paul met an expat who had worked in Asir for a year – where the architecture conference had taken place and ended badly. He said it was so conservative that in the entire year he lived there, he never heard a woman's voice or a woman's laugh. Let alone see a woman's face.

We took the students to an outdoor market and the stall owners, all women, were selling tradition Asiri crafts – large woven sun hats, baskets, wall hangings, small trinkets. As the girls milled around the stalls one women demanded to know where we were from. "Jeddah." I said. She harrumphed and tossed her covered head in the direction of the girls. "Why are they not covered?" she demanded. I didn't know what to say. They had on head scarves but we were in very conservative territory. I got a pass as an American. I shrugged, bought a trinket, and scurried away.

REFLECTIONS

Women, power, and the body were things I observed in Saudi society. In this small village were beautiful young women, completely covered except for the eyes where even a little movement to traditional music was frowned upon by the elder men of the village. History, society, governments, and marketing have tried to control women's bodies forever.

We buy into the false idea that we are not powerful, not empowered, or not beautiful. We carry this bias unconsciously into our adulthood and at some point, give up on trying to feel our best, since, after all it's too late and we're too old. SO not true!

The Grandmother of orphans in this village was beautiful, powerful, and empowered in her loving care and no doubt wisdom showered on the children without parents. I'm sure the last thing on her mind was her own level of fitness, she had a job to do and just did it. That gave her energy and purpose. She was giving service to others, but must clearly keep herself healthy in order to maintain this level of caring for young ones.

TO JOURNAL

- What gives you energy and purpose?
- Can changing your daily sedentary habits and nutrition give you more energy to give of yourself to the world?
- What small steps can you take now? Please remember, your loved ones and the world need you.

TWENTY-FOUR
WINDOWS TO THE SOUL

The first week I was in Saudi Arabia waiting for Paul's paper work to be approved I had a chance to go shopping outside the compound. Each Friday and Saturday, the compound bus took residents to one of the many mega-malls that were in Jeddah. It's a form of social contact and a way pass time – to stroll, shop, and buy the latest whatevers in a luxurious air-conditioned mall. The first time I went, I was completely put off by the faces I could not see. The women traveled in pods, some with children and nannies in tow; their faces were tiny and all looked alike.

I was determined not to feel shut out and would smile at them with my uncovered face. I covered my hair as was the custom but I was already an anomaly. But when I smiled and said in my passable Arabic,

"Peace be unto you, how are you?" (A salaam alaykim, keyf halek?)

I would see the eye corners crinkle and know a smile was under the niqab.

One time a small woman answered "Walakim Salaam" – which means peace be unto you too. Then she patted my arm and said Amreeeeka! No one ever said the United States. It was always America. Amreeka. If someone asked where you were from and you said the United States, we'd get a blank look until we said "America."

The paperwork to get Paul in the country was daunting. I had to go to a government office and the proper ministry to get everything signed and approved. Each office was gender segregated so I had to enter the side for women. One of the last papers to get was at a ministry downtown where a university driver dropped me off.

I went into the waiting room and faced a tall desk, similar to that of a police precinct. A sharp-looking Saudi official with a hook nose and black eyebrows over narrowed eyes gave me a stern look. He had on the traditional red checked head scarf, called a shemagh, and a crisp white thobe. I went up to the counter, but he motioned for me to sit down. There was a sign on the wall that said "Femail."

No one else was being helped. I sat with three other women who were clad completely in black. I don't know what business they had but after 30 minutes, this man must have decided I had sat long enough and curtly motioned for me to come forward. I gave him my paperwork and said I was there to get the signature for my husband to enter Saudi Arabia. Just then another official came behind the desk and they began to speak in Arabic and then laugh. Speak and laugh.

I had the feeling they were laughing at me. Finally, he said, "No, you need his passport copy!" Which was not true. But I left and came back the next day. The same ritual. I waited in the room for "femails" and when he was good and ready, he curtly motioned me forward. Acting tired and blasé, he held out his hand for the copy of Paul's passport, hit it a few times with a stamp, gave me another paper and said, "Khalas." (It's done.)

After Paul arrived and we exhausted our patience with drivers, we looked into buying a car. There were car dealerships everywhere and we decided on a new SUV for our dogs to be able to travel with us. We sometimes hiked out in the desert and had a friend take care of them when we traveled. Paul went into this dealership almost every other day for two months and came home with nothing.

When I asked what happened he said, "Nothing happened. I just sat there and no one really wanted to help me."

He would patiently wait until a salesman would come over and they'd discuss what was needed and he'd say nothing available, come back Thursday. This went on and on for two months! Meanwhile the guys there were getting to know Paul and like him. He was patient and kind to them and would just come back in a few days.

It was like they didn't want to sell any cars. In the U.S. if you walked into a dealership, you were walking out with keys to a new car. But this was Saudi Arabia.

Finally, we got somewhere. Paul's order was put in for the car, and the car actually arrived! I got a call from the dealership. A man said, "You can come now and get the car. Bring cash."

I told him we didn't have cash; we had a bank check. He said, "Okay, come anyway."

We arrived at the dealership, Paul said hello to one of his buddies who said, "Go on upstairs, the manager is waiting for you."

I had on my turquoise head scarf and when we entered the man's office he was in a suit and tie, sitting behind a big desk. He stood up and welcomed us and then looked at me and said, "You are very beautiful." I thought, *This guy has not seen a woman's face for so long except his wife's, a smiling American with a bright head scarf on would seem pretty cool.*

He invited us to sit down and asked us if we wanted some sweets. In fact, he had ordered a box for us as a gift to take when we left. Instead of talking about the car, he began to talk about his mother.

"You remind me of her," he said to me. "She and Allah were like this!" He held up two fingers intertwined in a tight embrace.

I couldn't imagine why I reminded him of his mother, but accepted the compliment; maybe she died when she was my age and that was frozen in his mind.

He told us he was Egyptian. Then he said, "You know when you go to sleep at night — I call it the 'little death' — and you meet people in your dreams and then you meet them out here?"

Then he looked at Paul and said, "Can I ask you a question?"

"Sure," Paul said.

"Are you Muslim?"

"No," Paul said.

"But I have watched you with my staff over these weeks." He then uncovered a hidden camera monitor near his desk that showed the sales floor. He had Paul on tape!

He said, "You have been so kind and patient with my staff, I thought this man is a Muslim."

After convincing him we were not Muslim, he opened the top drawer to his desk and took out a bottle of cologne. He raised the lapel on one side of his jacket spritzed his chest, then raised the other side for a spritz. He held it aloft and offered us a spritz. We shook our heads, "No, thank you."

"Well, you have the check?"
I handed it to him and he called his assistant to take us downstairs to the new car that was being prepped to leave the showroom.

"It was so nice to meet you. My wife is a teacher for the Quran, if your wife is ever interested in learning it," He told Paul.

We found throughout in Saudi Arabia that to convert a Westerner was the height of a Saudi's mission in life. We thanked him and left. I must say he completely charmed me and was really without guile. A genuinely sweet man.

We got in our new car and drove off.

REFLECTIONS

While living in Saudi Arabia, there was a freedom from focus on a woman's body. We covered up in an abaya, a form of robe that hid a woman's body. As a Westerner I was required to wear the abaya, but not always the head scarf, or tarha. One day I asked Paul to drive out into the desert to take pictures of me completely covered in a black abaya, head scarf, and niqab – the veil that is worn on the face with only slits for the eyes. I had some antique niqabs with beads and embroidery and I wanted to experiment with this in photography against the backdrop of the Arabian desert. No part of me was visible except my eyes.

As soon as I put on the entire ensemble, I felt a level of freedom and protection I had not expected. My physical identity was completely hidden. Even though it was just me and Paul out there in the desert, I felt deliciously invisible from the male gaze. It didn't matter AT ALL how I looked, whether I was wearing makeup, or had on my pajamas underneath. There was this incredible deep release from expectation from how a woman "should" look from a Western perspective. I was hidden. Hiding by choice. It felt freeing. I was shapeshifting.

You were born to SHAPESHIFT! It's in your nature as a human BEING.

We are so much more than who we are in this moment. We are a culmination of all the experiences we have ever had.

Experiences have wounded us, traumatized us, demoralized us. But these are the ones that have made us stronger.

Like lifting weights, you don't get stronger without resistance.

But before you get stronger you build protective strategies to cope.

Life has knocked us to our knees over the course of time. Each experience, no matter how grueling and devastating, can take on a patina of a real gift — OVER TIME.

Your health is a reaction to how you truly view yourself. Do you love you? Do you accept your amazing body the way it is TODAY?

Or do you hate aspects of it and constantly feed it negative self-talk when you look in the mirror?

Ask yourself what things you do to cope with those thingst hat are working against your health. You do have the answers in you or you could not ask the question.

Nanosecond mind shift away from the negative self-talk: Just thinking about what you're grateful for in your life can make anything that bothers you seem insignificant.

Find positive phrases to repeat to yourself. Because after all, you're amazing! BANG BANG!

Weight training, nutrition, and aerobic fitness are only part of the solution to feeling amazing – your mind has to work its magic, too. MINDSET MATTERS!

If you like to learn new things, dive deep into yourself and constantly SPIRAL UP. A fitness lifestyle is a perfect template to do so.

You think it's just about losing body weight?

That is the smallest part. There's a lot more inside that needs to be lost – psychological weight, toxic relationships, porous boundaries, negative self-talk.

CARRY ON!

TO JOURNAL

- What is your idea of beauty?
- On every level, what is beautiful about you?
- What coping mechanisms do you use that are working against your health?
- How can you change this in one small way this month?
- What positive phrases would be most helpful to you in your life right now?
- What other sort of weight do you need to lose that is not the body?

TWENTY-FIVE

OPPRESSION

When I moved to Saudi Arabia, I got to know the women in that culture on a very close level. I was invited to their homes for dinner, and interacted with them in the university, where they could take off the head scarf and abaya. Underneath they dressed just like any other college student in the U.S. or any other professional woman you would see in the world. The coverings were a protection against the male gaze and only men in their family were allowed to see them uncovered.

As anywhere, there were levels of being very strict and conservative or liberal about this. A woman's family – i.e., the father, set the tone. Brothers, uncles, husbands would adopt the same level of protection toward the women in their family – she must cover her face, or not, she must wear a head scarf always, or not. Many in the West see this as a control issue over the women, but I read it as an act of love and protection. Of course, there is always the extreme to this; usually, women would not have a lot of say in the matter – but more often than not, women would have a say – they could choose their marriage partner based on love, or not.

One of the most distressing aspects I experienced was from my American friends. "How can you go to Saudi Arabia?" they would ask. "Women are so oppressed there!" A few friendships ended due to this attitude. What I know is that women are oppressed in some way everywhere. It just looks different in Saudi Arabia. So, people with no knowledge of the culture paint that society with a broad brush based on untruths and bias. I heard a Saudi woman say once, "I don't want a white woman from the West telling me what is best for me – in covering or conducting my life. It is my life, not hers."

I consider the oppression my own mother experienced in her lifetime. Born in 1934, growing up during WWII, with three older brothers in combat. Her parents were consumed with their safety and the war. My mother got very little attention. In fact, it was very similar to what I experienced after my little sister died and my two baby brothers were born. I was no longer the focus, and felt I didn't receive concern, love, or attention. I didn't feel seen, heard, or cherished in my childhood mind. My mother probably had the same experience I did but was never able to unpack the feelings behind this that caused her to parent the way she did.

She was oppressed by society and what was expected of a young woman in the 1950s after the war. The baby boom was a symptom of all those veterans coming home to America and needing jobs and houses – buy, settle down, have a big family. She was in the middle of her college education when she met my father. The pressure to be married by age 21 was so great that she chose the path of marriage instead of following her dreams. It was not encouraged that women follow their dreams unless it meant husband, home, and babies. Obviously scores of American women felt this way, because the Baby Boom was created.

My mother's dreams included a college degree and a career in early-childhood education. It was not meant to be. It was a form of oppression that one does not see in any obvious way. It's hidden away in the heart, the longing to have a different life – or one where you have agency, choice, and empowerment and are applauded for your intelligence. She did not have that. She was admired for having six children, for her natural beauty, for her ability to get things done, organize, cook, and still have time to exercise with swimming and walking. I think she was so driven and it gave her so much excess energy, she had to do something. But it was perhaps her great painful secret. Unrealized dreams became a form of oppression. But we don't really see it, and women of that era didn't complain about it. So how is that different from women being oppressed everywhere? It's just another face of the oppression of women.

As I got to know and love my Saudi women friends, much of what we consider different in the culture became normalized. Within the context of living there, knowing individuals and loving them, it was clear as day that women everywhere want the same things but go about getting them differently.

This is where I believe as women that we have an opportunity to support, accept, and really understand our sisters around the globe. Especially those who are maligned in the media. It was a privilege to meet so many incredible women in Saudi Arabia who are still my dear friends.

Early, before things normalized for me, I had a student, Dima (not her real name.) She was sincere, intelligent, and very modern in her approach to life. She told me one day she was engaged. I was excited for her and asked his name. After she told me, I asked, "How did you meet?"

She said, "It was arranged."

She saw my face, and with a cocked head and tolerant smile as if indulging a child, added without apology, "That's how we do it in my country, Miss Julia."

Dima told me she had been taking Quran lessons with a well-known Imam (Islamic priest) who had given her a book to read. The book was about love, life, and serving Allah. After she read the book, the imam asked her if she liked it. She said yes, very much.

The Imam told her that the person who wrote it was a male student of his and he felt that he and she would make a strong marriage. Dima was open to the idea so her parents were brought in and they agreed to meet him. The boy came over to meet the father first, then the mother. As her parents waited, Dima was called into the room. I asked what happened then. She said, "I came into the room, met him, we talked a few minutes, had a few sweets, I said okay, I would marry him and he left."

Then the two families met and Dima and her fiancé were chaperoned every time they got together until the marriage happened. They had six months to get to know each other, during which time either party could call off the "engagement." The actual legal wedding was just between the two families and the Imam. A wedding party comes much later when the bride has her party, the groom has his — often on separate weekends — and they are gender segregated, with only women at hers, men at his. These weddings are ways for future mothers-in-law to suss out candidates for their sons. Women hold the power in the family in finding suitable brides for sons – alliances of families – and fortunes.

One young woman I'll call Ayesha, I met at work. She had been planning her wedding for a year. We all pitched in and got her a designer bag as a gift and took her to dinner a few weeks before the wedding. She was going to leave the job and her parent's house and move to Riyadh to live with her new husband.

Their story was different. They were in their late 20s, had known each other for more than 10 years and had been secretly seeing each other since they were 18. He wanted to marry her (18 is not young in Saudi Arabia for marriage) but she said no, she wanted him to get a degree and a good job and then she would marry him. Of course, this took years. All the while they were in a relationship neither set of parents had an inkling about.

The young man graduated with a degree, got a good job, so it was time. Ayesha was ready and happy to start a life with him out in the open as his wife.

Her beau went to his mother and said, "I saw this girl (it was Ayesha of course) and I would really like you to contact her mother and set up a meeting." He was signaling he was interested in marrying her – this is normal, but the boy will have never actually met the girl. He is interested in meeting her to see if it's a good match and she agrees.

I have another friend who had 39 of these kinds of proposals until she finally met number 40, and he was the one she accepted.

Ayesha's mother got the call from the boy's mother, a meeting was set up for both sets of parents. They brought their son over. Ayesha and her secret boyfriend had to act like they had never met before despite being in a relationship for almost 10 years.

The designer dress had been made, the invitations had gone out, gifts had been sent. Ayesha had quit her job. A week before the wedding, the boy called the whole thing off. He got cold feet. Ayesha was devastated. The boy's mother pleaded with Ayesha not to give up on him, but she was so crushed she only wanted to get away from the disaster.

For a Saudi woman's wedding (I was invited to several) there is lots of food, music, dancing, fancy gowns and jewels, and visiting. They happen very late at night in luxurious venues with female wait staff in special costume. The fragrant incense fills the air with scent. There is live music by male musicians who are projected on a large screen but sit in another banquet room performing. Hours go by as we wait for the bride to make her entrance.

Finally, the bride enters on the arm of her groom. It is usually around 2:00 a.m. and we are all advised to put on our hijabs before they appear. I would glance around and see 80-year-old wrinkly Saudi matriarchs cover their faces. It was tradition. But it's so all the women can get a good look at the new husband.

The boy would come in with his bride and look so scared. His mother and her mother would bring them to the cake, they would take a bite, then the couple would to sit up on stage or a dais to receive the men from the families who would parade in and go up and congratulate the couple. We remained seated and covered. Eventually after about 10 minutes all the men would leave, plus the groom, and we would eat and dance the night away. Just women, being women. It was gloriously fun! That was the night the wedding would be consummated – only after the parties had taken place.

The groom's party was a wilder affair – with traditional Saudi line dancing – and shooting off rifles and guns into the air. Our neighbor in Jeddah got married one evening after we moved in and I secretly watched the men arrive one by one to their large courtyard and go inside the private walled estate. The music started – a live band playing traditional Yemeni and Saudi music – and I could hear the raucous goings on but not see them.

Women in Saudi Arabia want the same things women everywhere want. Love. And they care about taking care of themselves. Under the black abaya – a tradition that is relaxing under the young crown prince – they want to be fit and feel healthy. There is a tremendous desire to be active – and they only recently were allowed to ride bikes in public. Many would go out in the desert and ride bikes away from the eyes of the religious police (who also have been disbanded under the crown prince). My husband Paul rode with many of these active cyclists who were women.

I felt a solidarity with women in that country – and felt the longing they had for different things than a woman from the West might want. But the longing was a feeling we all experience and attach importance to varied things we have available to us in life. It's different in every culture, but the hearts and incredible intelligence and power of women is evident everywhere in the world.

We had friends who had a weekend house up in the Tabuk region of Saudi Arabia - a six-hour drive through camel herds and desert, but on a good highway. We went up several times to stay with them – it was a town called Um Lujj or Um Lajj. It is directly on the Red Sea and in this area, which is undeveloped, the water is a brilliant turquoise. I have never seen anything like it! The water is crystal clear and the coast is dotted with small deserted islands you can boat out to. It's a magical, beautiful place. The crown prince has a palace on one of the bigger islands accessible only by boat. When he is there, you know from the yacht (I at first though it was a cruise ship – no, it's his yacht.) No boats are allowed to leave the harbor if he is in residence.

On one visit we took a tour of an old palace that had been turned into a series of art studios and exhibition spaces. We talked to the manager and I showed him my paintings and told him I taught art. I was invited to do a workshop for a week at the palace in this beautiful town of Umm Lujj. Our friends, a married couple with two boys – she's American and he is Saudi — helped me organize the workshop. The university also helped fund part of it and I crowd-funded the rest from friends in the U.S.A. I wanted to offer a drawing workshop for women alone; I had done the workshop so many times in Jeddah, and it was always a huge success.

As we planned the workshop, it was marketed by the palace manager. I could only take 20 students because of the size of the room – the slots quickly filled and ultimately there was a waiting list of more than 125 women who desperately wanted to take the drawing workshop. I was crushed I could not have them all.

I was then asked to provide a workshop for the men, too. It was segregated – men in the morning, women in the evening. It was double the amount of work, and I was not being paid. I was volunteering my time and resources, but it's what I loved to do. So, I agreed. I didn't want to charge for the workshop and with generous donations from many, I provided all the supplies and materials needed.

In that week I experienced a camaraderie that is hard to explain. In Umm Lujj you never see a woman with her face uncovered. There are no people from other parts of the world – rarely do they come through – so every woman that came was dressed in black from head to toe – only her eyes were showing.

Once we got started the head scarves and niqabs came off and it was a room of very engaged energetic women doing something new and exciting. I had a translator, as none of them spoke English.

Every night I would arrive for the workshop with the women and three or four would be standing outside begging to be allowed to come in and participate. But there was simply no way. It was so crowded, even with 20. After each evening I would have them tape their work to the wall on the right. And in the day, I would have the men tape their work on the left wall. In the morning the men would study the women's drawings and in evening the women would study the men's. They were doing the same exercises, and a fun rivalry was evident.

At the end of the week, I drew portraits of as many of the women as wanted me to – and gave them as gifts. I took pictures of the portraits they held up in front of their faces – Saudi women do not want their faces to be shown anywhere on social media.

I arranged an exhibition of all the work the men and women did and we had an art opening. Dignitaries from the local area came, articles were written in Arab media, and fathers of the girls came to see their daughters' work.

On the last day of the workshop, I was inundated with gifts from the women – beautiful drawings and paintings, jewelry, letters translated, and even a dress – in gratitude for the workshop.

Then the men came bearing gifts too – they had pooled their money and presented me with perfume and chocolates. I was so touched. It reminded me of the kind of gifts I would get from a boyfriend in junior high.

REFLECTIONS

I could travel the world doing these workshops in areas where women may not have opportunities to be creative and free – and do it 24 hours a day if this body could withstand it. It's because of my travels to so many countries that I feel connected to women all over the world. It doesn't matter the culture, the beliefs, the country, the physical characteristics of a woman – I feel a kinship.

I recall seeing a phrase once that said if you could read the full life story of a person, there is no one you would not love.

In this stage of my life, the kinship I feel is in the aging experience and how hard it can be for some women to navigate and live through. For me the answer has been fitness, which makes me feel ageless and energetic, with the strength I need to go after my dreams. One of those dreams is to empower women with the message that it is not too late, and you are never too old to get healthy and fit and glow with beauty from the inside out.

Find a word each week to focus on – that reflects a quality you need more of in your being.

FEARLESSNESS.
SOAR.
LOVE.
CALM.
STRENGTH.
ABUNDANCE.
RESILIENCE.

What do you need in your life right now?

Pick a word (or a phrase) that embodies it. Write it on a piece of paper, look at it every day for the week, feel it inside. Live it. See what happens. Take it into the next week, or keep it a month.

Thoughts can be so willy-nilly and blow with the wind. Having a focus and structure helps to reach goals because you're choosing thoughts that support your best life.

Like fitness, it is consistency and daily practice over time that will TRANSFORM you completely.

Does going to the gym one time make you fit? No.

Does going to the gym 208 times make you fit? YES, if you add nutrition goals too! 208 times – that's 4 days a week for a year.

If we want to transform on any level, we will find a way. If not, we will find an excuse.

TO JOURNAL

- How have your experienced oppression in your life?
- How has it made you stronger?
- Have you forgiven your oppressors?
- Write down a word or phrase to practice this week that will help you navigate life's challenges at this time or a quality you want to develop.

TWENTY-SIX

BURIED LIKE A KING

I could not live without my dogs and so taking Jabu and Bika to Saudi Arabia was a must. If they could not go, we could not go. But we found a way.

Bika had intense soulful eyes and she would look right into mine. Within a year of adopting her, she had a bowel obstruction from chewing up a piece of tennis ball. It lodged in her intestine, got infected, and burst. We were so vested in her as ours, there was no way we were going to let her go. We paid for the operation and it seemed after that she knew we would do anything for her. She was the most loving, loyal little orange girl.

Bika and I had such a closeness. I often said, "She was my heart." She was the female version of Tobe – she connected and bonded with us so deeply. Rescue dogs are so grateful – we had no idea of her prior life but she hit the lottery as one of our dogs. Friends would say that if reincarnation was real, they wanted to come back as one of our dogs.

Bika was 11 and Jabu was 7 when we moved to Saudi Arabia. After two years in Saudi, Bika's health began to decline.

She developed a strange cough, and was clearly aging. They both slept on beds next to ours and there were times she was in such a deep sleep, like she was so far away. If I roused her, she looked surprised to wake up until she saw me.

Bika began to significantly slow down and was suffering, getting worse by the day. We had Dr. Mohmmad, our Egyptian vet, look at her. Bika had congestive heart failure. I asked Dr. Mohammed if she had to be euthanized would he come to our villa for this?

He told me that vets in Saudi Arabia refuse to euthanize animals, because they feel taking life is the job of Allah only. But he could not see any animal suffer so he would agree to help her transition this way.

Around this time, King Abdullah, the monarch of Saudi Arabia, and one of the last sons of the original Monarch King Saud who founded Saudi Arabia, passed away. The country went into mourning. He was a well-loved king who championed women's rights, wanting them to get access to education.

His views were moderate and for many younger Saudis, this was the only king they had ever known. He was like a grandfather, as well as a father, to so many.

In Islamic tradition, within 24 hours King Abdullah was wrapped in a white sheet and buried in an unmarked grave. People remarked: "We come from Allah and to Allah we return." Then it was done and life moved on.

Bika was clearly in distress and declining fast. We didn't want her to suffer in any way or have a seizure or stroke – or die in pain. We arranged a time for Dr. Mohammed to come to our villa to help Bika transition. She was having a hard time breathing and coughing a lot and sleeping even more. I spent precious moments with her, cuddling and kissing her. She was reciprocal in affection but she was really struggling.

Dr. Mohammed arrived on the appointed afternoon, and began the procedure. He made her very comfortable with a sedative, making sure she had no feeling in her body before he stopped her heart. We let her rest for a long time and made sure she was in a deep sleep state from the powerful sedative – she was peacefully on her side on her floor pillow. I got down on the ground and Dr. Mohammed arranged the final shot. I hugged her sweet orange form with my lips to her head and whispered "I love you. I love you. My sweet girl. I love you, Bika."

As I held her, her heart stopped beating and she stopped breathing. Dr. Mohammed checked her heartbeat, which was no more.

"It is done," he said.

He had arranged to bury Bika on an Arabian Horse farm owned by a friend. By now it was dark and nighttime. We wrapped her in a white bedsheet and Paul carried her outside to Dr. Mohammed's car. He waited for him to pop the trunk.

"No, she will be in the backseat where my children sit. Not in the trunk." He was the most loving man.

He took her and gently placed her wrapped body in the backseat. We thanked him and he drove away. We went inside and wept.

There was relief mixed with grief, but just knowing she would not suffer anymore was a comfort.

In the morning I had a text message from Dr. Mohammed. It was a video. In it, a spotlight was shining in the dark onto a hole that two men were digging. They were intent on their work and were saying over and over: "Bismillah, Bismillah" – which in Arabic means in the name of Allah. "Bismillah" is said before any undertaking that is sacred or important.

They were saying it with so much reverence and respect. Then Dr. Mohammed appeared with Bika's body wrapped in the white bed sheet, and gently laid her in the grave they had dug. "Bismillah, bismillah bismillah." Then the video ended.

My Bika. My Bika. Buried with love and reverence like the King of Saudi Arabia. My Bika. I have a warm feeling in my heart knowing that my girl will always be in Saudi Arabia on the Arabian horse farm as her final resting place.

REFLECTIONS

Losses of many kinds become part of our life story as we move into our 40's, 50's, and 60's. Or they may happen sooner. But Queenagers have weathered a lot of life, which brings a certain wisdom and acceptance we extend to those around us that we love. But often, we weren't taught to extend that love to ourselves. This was my biggest lesson in getting healthy, I had to love myself enough to do it. It was an act of love, not something born out of self-loathing, or disgust with my body.

Because of my health challenges, I didn't have an expectation of living past 40. I had accepted the temporary nature of the physical body after my near-death experiences. It didn't make it easier to lose loved ones or beloved pets, but I still felt there was an expiration date looming for me somewhere in the future.

At age 62 in April 2019, as I began a fitness journey and got stronger and stronger, I no longer sensed that looming event somewhere in the future. I began to live my life in the present moment, savoring the boundless energy that exercise (lifting weights) and eating nutritious food gave me.

One day I stood in line behind a woman at the drugstore who was buying a bottle of wine. The cashier has to ask the birthday of the buyer of alcohol even though I could clearly see even from the back, with her white hair, she was over 21. I was shocked to hear her say the year she was born: 1927. I was 64 at that time and it hit me that she was 30 years OLDER than me!

I followed her to her car and respectfully said, "Ma'am, I'm sorry I overheard you say you were born in 1927. That's amazing!" She looked at me with sparkling blue eyes as she loaded her bags in the car, and said, "Yes, I'm 94 years old!" She was as energetic and full of life as a 20-year-old. I asked her what her secret was – she just shrugged her shoulders and smiled. I asked her if she exercised.

"Oh yes!"

"What do you do?"

"I sit and move my arms and legs around for 30 minutes every day." Her name was Eileen. If I live to be as old as Eileen I have at least 30 more years to go. I want to feel as good as she does.

Along the way, we have those times where we are just living our life and enjoying it. Our attention is on things other than being fit, but maybe we eat healthy and do sporadic exercise.

Then along comes that time, that you just know, things have to step up. CHANGE is needed. This happened in April, 2019 for me when my fitness journey began. I needed to be healthy. I had so much gratitude for still being alive at 62. So, I really dove in.

ENERGY FLOWS WHERE YOUR ATTENTION GOES. That's the path to TRANSFORMATION.

Time advances and our bodies wear a record of how we have treated it.

There may be no motivation to improve on it because we don't have role models like Eileen – we are invisible after age 50 – maybe sooner.

Older women are GORGEOUS. With it, comes the wisdom lines in the face, the clear sense of purpose in the aura, the empowered female energy.

Just kick ass amazing Queenagers.

Women are the ones who get it done. Raising families, caregivers for aging parents, dog and cat moms, CEOs, loyal workers day-in and day-out in all walks of life.

Let a life of giving turn toward YOU as you age. Give to YOU.

You have totally earned it, you amazing kickass QUEEN.

TO JOURNAL

- Describe yourself using the first 10 words that come to mind.
- Then, list 10 words that you'd *like* to use to describe yourself.
- List a few ways to transform those descriptions into reality.
- Where do you want to be in 10 years?
- How does it feel to look that far ahead?

- What three things would you most like others (loved ones, potential friends and partners, professional acquaintances, etc.) to know about you?

TWENTY-SEVEN

SOMEONE DIES AND
SOMEONE LIVES

When I was 17, I'd had enough of diabetes. After six years of living with it, I desperately wanted to be healed of its wretchedness. I read about spiritual healing and wondered if God would grant me such a miracle. I prayed fervently – to be healed of diabetes.

I was chanting HU and asking for this healing every day. I was sincere and open. During one of these prayer times, this inner message came, definitive and loving, from somewhere beyond me: "You will be healed."

I was startled, but it was unmistaken what I'd heard.

I inwardly asked, "How? How will I know?"

The answer was just as clear:

"You'll wake up one morning and it will be gone."

I was instantly at peace. I surrendered my worry and care about a healing to God and with a great sense of calm went on with my life. Every day wondering if this was the day. Would I wake up and it would be gone? I truly believed the message I had gotten during my prayers.

Life went on and my health actually got worse, instead of better. I forgot about my prayer, my plea and the answer I got during the HU chanting.

Seventeen years after that prayer, and two years into my marriage to Paul, I began to feel unusually sick. I had stopped going to doctors for a while. I felt like I knew more than they did and nothing was out of whack. Until it was. I was tired all the time and felt nauseated and lifeless. It was confirmed: My kidneys were finally failing. I was 34 years old.

It was an event in a long line of diabetic complication events – retinopathy of the eyes that cause blindness, neuropathy (nerve damage), and now kidneys failing. It was February of 1991.

The previous November I had a dream that I wrote down in my journal. It was a very lucid dream. I was holding a black-and-white photo of myself surrounded by people dressed in white – like the event had already happened. We all looked happy. I didn't recognize anyone. The most striking feature of the dream was a living, six-pointed, golden-white star pulsating at my forehead. It was in the area of what some say is the spiritual eye.

In addition, there was a diffused, less bright light hovering near my right pelvic hip bone. I awoke feeling so happy and peaceful but had no idea what the dream meant. I wrote it down but almost didn't include the diffused light at my right side. It seemed so dim compared to the one at my forehead.

I forgot about the dream.

After the February appointment with the nephrologist, he explained what my options were. Dialysis – which would need to start in eight weeks. This could give me five to six more years of life as a diabetic on dialysis. Or a kidney transplant from a living donor or cadaver donor, with dialysis keeping me going until one was found. We met with the transplant team at the university hospital where surgery would take place. The lead transplant surgeon had worked with the pioneers of organ transplantation in Pittsburgh. It was explained he was also doing experimental pancreas transplants for patients who were diabetic and needed a kidney. Both the pancreas and the kidney would have to come from a cadaver donor.

Only about 2,000 of these had been done, with varying success, but results were hopeful overall. In my case, I also had heart disease. But at age 34, I was relatively young and in good health, compared to some of the sicker patients they saw. I was considered a good candidate for both. However, there were risks. I could die during the operation, after the operation, or have a stroke or heart attack at any time. Being under anesthesia for that amount of time was also a risk – 11 to 12 hours for both, half for just the kidney. But if just the kidney were transplanted, I would still have diabetes. The choice was mine to make. Paul also said the same – he could not make the choice for me. I had to decide myself.

We'd only been married for two years and it was like finding my lost love. When we walked down the path in our outdoor wedding, the feeling was this: I have found "THE ONE."

We got home and I went upstairs to our bedroom to chant HU and just think. I mindlessly picked up my journal and flipped through a few pages until it fell on the dream from November. The light at my forehead and right hip area. My answer of what to do was there in black-and-white: my handwriting. The light at my side was the exact location the doctor said he would put the pancreas. I felt it was a prophetic dream to help me know the right choice when the time came. I let the transplant team know my decision. I would go for both organs.

I began to wear a beeper – no cell phones yet – and awaited a call from the hospital that they had a donor. Every week my blood was taken to be tissue typed and make sure I got a good match. I was still working but having to lie down every hour to rest. My weight plummeted and I did not feel good. I was weak and had no muscle tone. It was a waiting game with huge ramifications.

As I passed people on the street, at work, or in stores, I wondered – *Who will my donor be?*

I was basically waiting for someone to die – and it gave great poignancy to every person I saw or encountered. They might be the one, this precious person. What does life hold for any of us at any moment? For me, the possibility of life into advanced years without diabetes. For someone else, my organ donor, an end to life.

By July I was in really bad shape as my kidneys had almost completely failed. It was time to ready me for dialysis. I could wait a long time for a donor. I was on the wait list at UNOS (United Network of Organ Sharing) which shared allocated organs based on geographic location and patient need. I went into outpatient surgery on Friday, July 26 so they could go into my left wrist, pull up a deep, large artery from my arm and bring it to the surface and create a fistula. This helps getting blood in and out of the patient's bodies for the cleansing of blood that dialysis provides. The kidneys no longer filter the toxins.

Paul took me home after that surgery and I went to bed. It was a beautiful summer night. That very night at 2 a.m., the phone rang in our hallway. I was super annoyed – who the hell would be calling at this hour? Paul answered and spoke softly so I could not hear. He came back to the bed and said, "That was Barb, the transplant coordinator. They have your organ donor." The crickets were singing outside the open window. The dark leaves on the trees I could see from the bed caught a little light from the street lamp.

I quickly sat up in the bed and wondered about another family somewhere, we didn't know where, who was mourning as we at the same time faced a future of health for me – possibly. We said a prayer for them and got dressed to take a walk in our small town. There was no going back to sleep. A police car drove by and I said, "What will we tell them if they ask why we're out? They will never believe us."

We got to the hospital. I called my parents from the pay phone in the hospital lobby. I started crying. I was the little kid again, needing their love and support. They would be on their way as soon as the sun came up. But there were hours of prep, taking blood samples, getting IVs inserted, signing papers before I'd be rolled into the operating room. What did the future hold for me?

A year before I knew that I was going to need an organ transplant I had a prophetic feeling that I was going to die, soon. It wasn't based on my state of health at that time, which had not been identified as being in jeopardy, but I just thought the expiration date was coming. It made me sad on the deepest levels because Paul and I had been married only a year. I had finally found him, but it was so soon to be over.

251

I carried this feeling of loss and dread so deep that I could not speak of it.

Finally, when I got on the waiting list for the transplant, I shared this prophetic feeling with Paul. "I feel like I'm going to die."

Paul was quick to say, "I felt this coming from you, but I know that you will be okay. I know that everything is going to be okay." He sounded so sure. I wasn't convinced. But what turned out to be a death was the "old me." Sickly, diabetic, weak and tired – she was going to "die" and a new me was going to emerge.

Sometimes the "old" us really has to leave.

REFLECTIONS

For every woman who has felt inadequate, small, worthless, over the hill, old, past their prime, ugly, fat, sick and tired of being sick and tired....

No matter how you got to that thought – it stops right now. If a family member, friend, doctor, or your own negative self-talk is telling you this, it's not the truth. It stops. NOW.

Because you are never too old for anything and it's never too late! As long as you are breathing, you have life and tomorrow is another day to manifest your heartfelt dreams.

You have to start somewhere. Quit telling yourself it's overwhelming. Quit convincing yourself you don't know where to start. Quit waiting for someone to do it for you. EMPOWER you. You are a complete package of wisdom and energy – that person inside of you that wants to come out in all her badassery, get in touch with her. Listen to that still small voice, what she's been trying to tell you.

You can't live your best life if you don't feel good. I so totally get that. It's ingrained in my being because of my health challenges early in life – being so close to death because my body was about to give up and just stop working.

TO JOURNAL

- Do you need to say good-bye to the "old you" so that the "new you" can emerge?
- What special ritual might you design to make this a loving gesture of expanding into your Best Life and Best Self?
- What does your best self look like? Write down where you will be in a year from now.
- What is the badass woman inside of you trying to tell you?

TWENTY-EIGHT
THIS WAS THAT MORNING

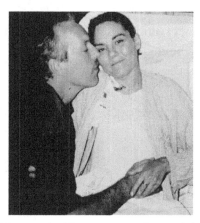

July 27, 1991 - post double organ transplant with husband Paul

My parents had come to our wedding with reservations. In fact, they were tough on Paul when they first met him. My father in particular. He challenged Paul's motives on his first visit to Indiana to meet them. It was after the Atlanta conference where I realized I was totally in love. I called my parents and asked if I could invite a friend for Thanksgiving. I planned to go, and Iowa was not far from Indiana. A good time to meet my family.

My parents said, sure, that's fine.

I added:
"His name is Paul. I'm in love with him and I'm quitting my job in New York and moving to Iowa to be with him."

Dead Silence.

Later, I realized that since we had been together more than a year in pure friendship, I had not mentioned Paul to my parents. He was "just a friend" to me. Nothing to talk about. When things so quickly changed, they had never heard his name and never heard the back story, nor were they interested in it. All they knew was that my first husband Sam had been abusive and that lasted 10 months. What is she getting herself into now?

It was an awkward Thanksgiving. My dad having the man-to-man talk downstairs, challenging Paul. I was aghast. Worse than the phonies at the party in New York City. Our wedding was held in a wood-lined park and was fairly small with about 40 friends and family. My parents came, but my father did not give me away, as he did the first time. I didn't think he wanted to, so I didn't ask.

Lauren, Paul's daughter, was our ring bearer. My brother played a classical piece on his guitar, and the cleric did a beautiful ceremony. Afterward, we had a party in our backyard under the trees, with a four-piece string band, grilled meat, and lots of other food. Paul and a close friend had picked wildflowers out in the country for each table that day.

Two years later when I went to the hospital for the transplant, things changed for my parents and Paul.

Finally, the time came to go into the operating room. I was prepared medically, but my parents had not yet arrived. Paul followed me behind the gurney with my medical team down the long white hallway to the surgical ward. The doors that led to the operating room swung open to more doors with big black numbers on them. Mine had 14 on it.

They stopped the gurney so Paul and I could have a moment. I didn't know if I was going to see the face I loved ever again. He had kept telling me it was going to be okay – but I knew because I had no fear of death – "everything being okay" would be true either way, even if I didn't physically survive.

I took his love into the operating room with me and he released me into their care.

It was 1:00 p.m. when I was rolled me into operating room #14. There was my transplant surgeon at a table handling what looked like chicken fat in a stainless-steel pan. He looked at me over his mask and I could see the excitement in his eyes. He was handling the organ in the pan like it was the most precious jewel in creation. Our eyes met – I saw great hope in his. His eye corners crinkled, and I smiled back at him.

The room was full of nurses and anesthesiologists and everyone was bustling about like it was a party. The atmosphere was positively charged – this was a rare event. An experimental double organ transplant – a kidney and a pancreas — on a childhood-onset diabetic, age 34, with severe complications. All the medical professionals were excited to be there. Three surgeons, medical residents, medical students, nurses. It was crowded but it was a big room. I knew they were all there for me. I was the guest star at this party.

The anesthesiologists had on green scrubs and safety glasses. There were three and they bent over me like praying mantises. One explained what they would be doing to put me out.

"Who will I see last?" I asked.
"All of us."
"Would you say a phrase for me when you put me out?"
"Sure, what's the phrase?"
"There is only God's Love."
"Let me write that down."
One of the anesthesiologists went and grabbed a pencil and I thought what is a lead pencil doing in the OR? Isn't lead dangerous?
I said it again for him.
"There is only God's Love."
Scribbling it down he asked,
"Will this phrase help me pass my medical board exams?"
I said, "It will further your career!" We laughed.

Then it was time.

I have no recall of the next 12 hours. I feel like I went somewhere very far away for a very long time. At 2:00 a.m. I was awakened by someone screaming "It hurts! It hurts!"

A nurse was saying something to me but I couldn't hear her. She raised her voice to a yell, "Julia! Your husband is here!"

I snapped out of it and realized I had been the one screaming. I saw Paul's face and knew I had survived the operation. I looked at him and said "I love you!"

When I awoke after surgery in the ICU, I immediately knew my body was healed and that the surgery was a success, despite the pain.

I was lucid enough in that moment to be hit with a reality and a promise I had carried with me since I was 17. The prayer for healing from diabetes. The answer that was that I would just wake up one morning and the diabetes would be gone.

This was that morning.

It has been the greatest gift of my life to have received a cure for childhood diabetes through an organ transplant. I would not have lived to 40 otherwise. To receive a working kidney from a donor who was almost a perfect match to me.

The doctors said the blood and antigen match was so close we could have been sisters. Suddenly my life opened up to decades ahead to enjoy life with Paul and find ways to honor this gift.

My organ donor's name was Gina. She died in a car accident in Colorado. She was 25 and married and had moved to the mountains, which she loved. She also loved wooly worms as a child and named them – two in particular, Fred and Ethel – and her mother told me she was so healthy and excited about her new life in Colorado.

She was born late to her parents and had two older siblings. In 1991, you were not allowed to meet your donor family – letters were sent through hospitals with no last names or any identifying information for contacting. These days, donor families and recipients can meet if both agree.

Gina's mother's letters stopped after about five years and mine were returned – address unknown. I figured her parents had died.

With the thirtieth anniversary of my transplant coming up I wanted to try again to be in touch with my donor family. She had siblings and a husband – I needed to write a letter of deepest gratitude to whomever is left. After God, and my parents, Gina's gift gave me life, the gift of life. It could have turned out so much differently.

When I awoke after the 12-hour surgery, I could tell without a doubt that my body was working. I felt the same easy flow of vitality and life force that I did at age 10 before I became diabetic. I still have the print out showing how the kidney and the pancreas worked right away after hook up. My creatinine level went from 6.0 to .9 and my blood sugar stabilized at 95. It was truly miraculous.

After being in intensive care, I was in the hospital for two more weeks. It was mid-August, and summer was in full bloom. Paul wheeled me out to the rooftop garden at the hospital. There were several huge cement containers spilling with colorful summer flowers. I looked out across the flat Iowa landscape beyond the town into the horizon of green corn fields. The sky was so deep blue it looked dark. White clouds were moving almost imperceptibly, across that blue dome. I burst into tears at the beauty – so green and lush, the sky, the clouds, the flowers and their intense colors. I had not noticed life around me in so long. I had been sick for a long time, just trying to survive day to day. Nothing else got my attention but how awful I felt. It was truly the first time I felt alive in so many months, and the first time I felt healthy since childhood. My joy was returning.

When my parents arrived at the hospital I had been in surgery for an hour. My mother was beside herself at the prospect of losing another child. It was very hard for her. She came into the ICU the next day and put her hand on my arm but could not speak. I felt her tears dripping on my arm. ICU visits were short. My parents left that afternoon.

What they went away with was a newfound respect for Paul. During all of this time, on the waiting list, during my sickness, he was my rock. He was cheery and positive and responded to my every need, my every concern. He was calm, steadfast, caring, and gentle.

My parents arrived at the surgical waiting room in such a highly agitated state. And there was Paul – tall, green-eyed Paul – calm, open, warm, and assuring them it would all turn out well. I don't think they could have loved him more during those hours. Their respect and love grew for him the longer we were married. They could see his devotion, deep love, and unending support for their daughter.

Once I was home and settled into a new routine, and it was clear my body had accepted Gina's organs, I called Dr. Mirsky in New York. He was dear to me. In those days you could get the doctor on the phone. I asked to speak to him, and said, "Dr. Mirsky, this is Julia Linn. I just wanted to call and tell you that I've had a kidney and pancreas organ transplant and the diabetes has been cured."

He didn't stop to congratulate me, he simply yelled over the phone receiver to his staff: "Julia Linn had an organ transplant and her diabetes is cured!" I could hear applause in the background. I was sure they wouldn't remember me, but he did. They shared in his exuberance at my news. Then he came back on and congratulated me. I wish there were more Dr. Mirskys in the world.

REFLECTIONS

Our bodies are simply amazing. What mine has gone through and continues to serve me in a life that is full of energy and zest for living is incredible to me. But I have honored this body beyond anything I have ever done in my 7th decade of life. From age 62 to now. Knowing my 30-year anniversary of the organ transplant was coming up in two years, spurred me into action. I had to do something to really take care of this body, the Chariot for the Soul, and on a much bigger scale, a higher level, a huge SPIRAL UP.

Our bodies are designed to want to be healthy, strong, and alive. Think about how quickly a cut will begin to heal (in minutes!) or how the body heals from any kind of trauma or broken bone, surgery, or illness. It's always seeking HEALTH. And yet we ply it with junk food, and never actually take really good care of it in the way that's needed. As decades roll by, it begins to show in heart disease, cancers, diabetes, high blood pressure, obesity.

But it will immediately start to heal if we apply self-love, self-care, and are consistent with exercise and nutrition. It starts with your mindset, and your spirit – how badly do you want to be healthy and fit?

Your body is the most precious possession! But ... you are so much more than your body.

Thoughts and experiences like my organ transplant give me reason to be grateful and ready for everything I can do to keep my health in stellar condition. Bodybuilding and excellent nutrition has been the sustainable answer for me.

The inside stuff: mindset, consciousness, spirit – is just as connected. It's a feedback loop, a full circle that offers precise results if you can learn patience.

TO JOURNAL

- Write a love letter to every part of your body you have spent time hating. Tell this body part all the things you appreciate it has done for you and continues to do for you. Each part has a job to perform to keep your Chariot going so you can live life.
- What simple everyday physical actions have you experienced the loss of during an illness or injury?
- What are your thoughts on aging? Do you fear it or do you feel resigned to it?
- Make a list of the negative thoughts or beliefs you hold about aging. Think about each one and where it came from. Then cross it out and make an empowering statement from your inner warrior, your Queenager Shapeshifter inside who is ageless.

TWENTY-NINE
WOMEN SUPPORTING WOMEN

Whenever I have wanted to change something in my life, I knew I had to change my thinking first. I had to change what was in agreement with me deep down – the things that I believed to be true and how this fueled the thoughts that went through my being. Not just my mind, but my heart and soul. Thoughts are fleeting and ephemeral and can go in a million different directions and pivot on a dime into something you did not anticipate.

Ever get bad news? Or good news? Notice how your thoughts explode into a new area when something outside of you confirms a blessing or a loss. It can happen so fast.

My belief is that we create our lives in this plastic universe which is moldable by the thoughts we think and what we hold constantly in our hearts as being true. The universal, divine energy – the atoms of God if you will —, fill that mold we make with our thoughts, feelings, desires, and beliefs and in time the reality out here catches up and we have manifested it ourselves.

We are co-creators with life. Our life. Either knowingly or unknowingly. This universal divine energy does not care which it is, it just responds because we are creative beings – and it is our birthright to create a fully expressed life. And whether we are conscious of doing it or not – it will manifest.

There is a time lag for this to manifest "out here" and usually we give up way too soon. Let the pieces on the chess board be moved in the divine strategy of immutable spiritual law.

My goals and dreams early on were mostly about self-fulfillment and doing what I loved. Later what became more important was and is sharing with others what I have learned from what I have gone through.

There's great power in humans sharing their stories and struggles. We lift each other up, inspire and give hope. So many have done that for me.

When I was on the waiting list for an organ transplant, I had a tremendous amount of fear. I didn't know how it was going to go and I was in limbo-land. I had already had a near-death experience. I experienced a reality and life outside of my physical body so I knew that was not really *me* — that something else was really me – my spirit, or me as Soul. Soul (not *my* soul, but me *as* soul) was having a human experience.

So, the thought I might die before, during, or after the organ transplant was *well, it might happen.* I truly felt like I was going to die and that made me sad because Paul and I had just found each other and married two years prior. We had not had a chance to spend our lifetime together and I wanted to grow old with him. I knew that might not happen.

Paul was also having his own thoughts about this and continually told me, "I know everything is going to be okay. You are going to be okay."

That was not an iron-clad promise of anything because even if I left this body permanently, I knew I was going to be okay. There was life after this body – no doubt at all, because I had experienced the reality of that.

All of the experiences I've had with my body have shown me the connection between our thoughts, feelings, and purpose of our lives. I don't know your purpose and sometimes don't even know if I am hitting mine, but I do know there is a sacred pact of some kind that we fulfill in this life using our unique talents, skills, and beingness. It's a kind of blue print. We all know when we are not heeding the blueprint; at least I do. It's taken me so many years to gain the wisdom from all the struggles I've had. Every difficult thing has been a golden opportunity to be more aware and move into what author Gay Hendricks calls our "Zone of Genius." Doing what we love and are meant to be doing in this life.

When women share their struggles, it can inspire someone else to feel "I can do this too!" Like Roger Bannister, the 25-year-old medical student from Britain, who ran the first four-minute mile. Once he did it, others were able to reach that milestone. The mind is the only thing that holds back the triumphs we look for.

When I was on the waiting list for an organ, yes, I feared not living to see old age with Paul. But I was not afraid of dying. I saw an article during that time about a woman who was an early double organ transplant recipient. Former childhood diabetic. Complications. Kidney and pancreas transplant. Just like me. She looked healthy, as if she were functioning well. She even looked a little like me. If she could do it, I knew I could, too. I can still picture her in my mind. It gave me tremendous hope.

While living in San Francisco in 2005, I was teaching one day and couldn't catch my breath. I could feel air going into my lungs but I felt like I was suffocating. The shortness of breath indicated that my heart disease had advanced and it was time to see a heart surgeon. They did a cardiac catheterization and said my arteries were too small for a stent. I would need a triple cardiac bypass. The very thought of that made my stomach turn.

One of my close friends, a surgeon I met during my transplant after-care, was married to a heart surgeon. I sent Tony my films to get a second opinion. He knew my history and me as a person. I needed to know if the heart surgeon in San Francisco was correct.

Tony assured me I needed one and told my heart surgeon, "She'll be back."

I kept putting it off trying alternative methods of healing. I looked into chelation therapy where the arteries are cleansed of plaque. I studied Dr. Dean Ornish's diet – anything to avoid the bypass. I would stand in front of the bathroom mirror and run my hands between my breasts and down the breast bone, thinking, *They will saw me in half right here.* I couldn't bear it and wondered what the scar would look like.

As I procrastinated, I was home one day and had a crushing pain in my chest. Due to nerve damage, diabetics usually don't have the heart pain or angina a normal person would with a heart attack. Women also have different heart attack symptoms than men; such as nausea and shortness of breath.

I called Paul at work and said, "You're not going to like what I'm about to say but I think I'm having a heart attack."

He told me to call 911 and he was going to send Jeff over, his friend and colleague, since he was physically the closest person to our house. Paul was in the city working. Jeff came, and looked completely stricken — like if I died right there, he would be forever guilty of not doing anything. The ambulance came and loaded me in and we sped off to the ER. As I waited to be seen by the cardiac team, a small Filipino nurse came into the room and said, "Dear, what are you in for?"

I said, "I think I'm having, or had, a heart attack."

"They'll be here in one minute, don't worry." She was so soothing and sweet.

I said, "They want me to get a triple bypass, but I'm scared to have it done."

She looked at me with compassion. "Why, my dear?"

"I don't want to be sawed open."

She wordlessly opened the top of her nursing uniform and showed me a pink scar that ran down her chest and disappeared into the uniform.

She gently said, "See? I've had one done. It's not a big deal. I am back to work for some time now. "

In that moment, I had a nanosecond mindshift. If she can do it, so can I!

Within days I called the heart surgeon and said "Okay, let's do it."

When I awoke from cardiac surgery I was again screaming, "It hurts, it hurts!" The same as after the transplant but I don't remember anything, other than being very agitated. Paul was completely alarmed as they kept giving me morphine and it was not making a difference. I don't remember this at all. I do remember being in a lot of pain. I didn't have the same miraculous feeling of healing that I did with my double organ transplant. Someone had sawed me open, and another human being had handled my actual heart organ. They took an artery from my right leg and another from my chest and fashioned clean arterial bypasses around the diseased arteries of my heart.

Handling the human heart, I learned, can be extremely hard on the mental state of the patient, for up to two years. If the patient is put on a heart-lung bypass machine, their heart is stopped while the surgery is performed – it that can be worse. You are clinically dead for the duration of the surgery.

My surgeon was skilled in doing the "beating heart" bypass where my heart was not stopped. I was not on the heart-lung bypass machine, and my heart continued to beat on its own during the surgery. Still, I was depressed for the next two years, not my normal state.

REFLECTIONS

With all the trauma my body has gone through, I've learned to be patient with its cycles of healing and disease. The body will do its thing and sometimes all we can do is love and care for it. Being angry at my body or disgusted with my body was my mindset as a young person. That this body has persevered through all the medical adventures is amazing to me. In my fitness journey, what I came with was to allow the body its natural rhythms and cycles.

It took me four months to lose ten pounds, but my goal was health and vitality, not bathroom scale victories. I allowed my body the time it needed to adjust to my new lifestyle because it was never going to go back to the "old way" of non-activity and unconscious eating habits.

REFLECTIONS

Did you ever have a "gut feeling" about something? That's your body intelligence.

You are a broadcasting tower radiating energy and magnetically pulling people, circumstances, and ideas to you – but you are also a mystical genius. Meaning you know more than you know. Your body is an instrument that has wisdom & intelligence.

Learn to LISTEN TO YOUR BODY! Learn to LOVE YOUR BODY!

I was so good at listening to my body as a childhood diabetic, so vigilant about my blood sugar levels – I could give the exact reading without even testing it. After my double organ transplant, which cured the diabetes, my body intelligence grew.

And here's what loving my body did for me.

I woke up in the Intensive Care Unit from a 12-hour surgery and had someone else's organs in my body (Gina's, God bless her!) The diabetes was immediately cured and I had a working kidney. A miracle!!!

But within a week, my body recognized the invaders and began to reject the organs. I was given huge doses of anti-rejection meds via IV which caused extreme chills and fever. They called it "shake and bake!" Rejection averted!

From that day on, I gave Gina's donated organs all my love, every day, targeting them with my gratitude. I imagined love, a pure stream of white light and sparkly, soothing music wash over them. Every day.

I still do this. Her organs are mine now. They were, from the first moment.

I had to allow my body intelligence to know it was OK. They were not invaders. I love those "babies." I have never had another rejection episode.

And I bless Gina every day.

If that doesn't show the power of LOVING YOUR BODY, I don't know what else does.

Except this: start weight training, fuel your body with clean food, get enough sleep, and prioritize your health.

Forget the scale, use a tape measure, watch your fat go, your muscles come, and best of all you'll feel AMAZING!

Not just in BODY, but MIND & SPIRIT too! ♡

Life is a miracle, y'all!

But you already knew that.

TO JOURNAL

- When have you listened to a "gut feeling" and acted on it?
- Do you ignore gut feelings or how your body actually feels?
- List and describe five ways your body tells you something important.
- Do you act on those messages?
- When has it been a challenge?
- When has the outcome been positive?

THIRTY

TRANSFORMATION

When I turned 62, nearing my 30-year anniversary of being healed of diabetes due to the double organ transplant, I felt such gratitude for the added years. Open heart surgery also extended my life. Despite having my thyroid removed at age 50, my body was working just fine, but I was out of shape, tired, sluggish. This love for life and joy switched on in me and I thought – I have to take care of this body! It's so precious. I want optimal health, strength, vitality, energy — and yes, muscles!

Until then, I was sporadic about working out. In Saudi Arabia, I took advantage of the gym where we lived. My husband Paul inspired me to keep working out when in 2017, he rode his bike from Amsterdam to Florence, Italy. Almost 2,000 kilometers, 32,000 feet of elevation – over the Alps! – at age 65. I stayed in Saudi and used GPS to track his progress and book Airbnbs along his route. I am incredibly proud of his accomplishment. He went solo and carried only what he had on his bike.

In 2019, my Saudi Arabian teaching contract ended, I was offered another professor position in Mexico so we moved. It was there that the fire was lit to get fit. I took on a fitness challenge, got involved in an online group for accountability and camaraderie. After 12 weeks I won the fitness challenge.

My body had tightened up, I felt amazing, my inches were down, my weight was down. I had such energy! But then it stalled. I looked for the next phase – and found an in-person coach who owned a gym to take me to the next level of fitness. I made great strides in getting leaner and stronger. He suggested I enter a body-building competition. I asked him, "What's that?"

He explained how different age groups of women in different divisions show off their hard work in the gym on stage, in a bikini.

Me? At age 63? I was incredulous, thinking, *Who wants to see a 63-year-old woman on stage in a bikini?!* But I was intrigued by the idea and the goal. My coach could see how hard I worked in the gym. But then the Covid pandemic hit and the gyms closed.

I was so invested and loving the fitness/body building lifestyle that I had to continue. But I know you need to learn from those who know. I didn't want to flail on my own. I found a coach online and began to work with her. She was a contest prep coach – helping athletes get ready for competitions and the first thing she said to me was – "Find a competition and tell me by Monday which it is and give me the date."

My motto became "day-in and day-out" to drive home one of the keys of success in fitness – repetitive positive actions – lifting weights day-in and day-out. Consistency, time and patience.

The biggest aspect of this ongoing experience in fitness is how I have transformed on the inside. What I have learned about myself, the way my life has prepared me for such goal-setting and success in this endeavor. When I'm asked, "How did you do it?" I sometimes say, that would take a book. This is that book.

I worked with my prep coach for six months and on June 26, 2021, almost 30 years after my double organ transplant, and 16 years after my triple cardiac bypass, and 14 yeares after my thyroidectomy, I stepped on the stage in my sparkling turquoise bikini at the Orlando Sheru Classic NPC Masters Bikini 55+ Contest and won First Place. I was so thrilled to be on stage, and meet such amazing fitness people. I didn't care that I was the only competitor in my age group – and that I won by default! I showed up. I did the work. I started 26 months ago and transformed my body. I also won fifth place for True Novice – a class for women who have never competed before, all ages.

The following weekend, in Charleston, SC, I again stepped on the stage, this time for the NPC Masters Bikini 60+. I had two competitors – who quickly became my friends. I was honored to share the stage with them and placed third. I was the oldest of the three of us at 64. I felt like I won just being there!

In this fitness lifestyle, an enviable body is a shallow goal. My goal is to express my gratitude for life and the ability to move my body and be healthy for the rest of my days. My priority is to make sure that I can give back to my loved ones, that I can serve in my life, that I can live my life with joy and energy and vitality and honor my organ donor Gina, for giving me a second chance at life. My life is a miracle! (So is yours, by the way!)

Having an enviable body was never on my list of priorities. Whether or not I have one doesn't matter. I feel amazing and have no physical limitations. I love going after goals – like competing in an NPC Bikini Masters Competition at 64. Women in their 60's often feel it's over. Honey, it has just begun!

My gratitude for life is in every breath I take. That I can get out of bed in the morning and walk, breathe easily and be involved in life, is like winning the lottery. There were years, months, and days where I could barely manage to move – because diabetes robbed me of my life force early. Contending with the complications was harrowing but after the transplant, they lessened or reversed altogether.

I never felt safe or secure when I had diabetes. The high blood sugars did the damage but the low blood sugars – the hypoglycemia — was the worst. It would begin by white spots in my vision then I would feel shaky and anxious and eventually I couldn't talk. If I tried to tell someone I was having an insulin reaction I could not get the words out and I would just cry. If I did manage to get the words out – "I need sugar" – if someone knew I was diabetic and didn't understand diabetic hypoglycemia, they would say – "But you are not supposed to have sugar, right?" I did not have the wherewithal to explain in that moment.

Once the hypoglycemia was corrected the blood sugar would rebound and then remain high for a day – there was never a balance. I found that sunburns caused my blood sugar to go up to dangerous levels because of the cortisol it released in the body. Stress did the same.

In all these experiences I got to know my body. I stopped blaming it for not being what I wanted it to be. I learned to be at peace with whatever happened and to do my best in every moment. I also learned compassion for others who were suffering with bad health or debilitating disease because I myself knew what it was like. The body has intelligence. I learned to listen to it. More importantly, I learned to love it.

All parts of my being are involved with transformation. My spirit, mind, body. The inner work shows up on your body. The body is a metaphor for your inner state.

We can live years without focusing on our bodies. We can ignore it and look up one day and say who the hell is that? How did I get so out of shape? As a child, I was forced to focus on my body and it brought challenges. Like many women, I grew up concerned with how I looked, my weight, did I fit in, was I good enough, pretty enough, thin enough.

As I aged, I started being grateful for my body's resilience despite devastating chronic illness. I looked past the bloated belly, dowager's hump, flabby batwings, and lumpy thighs. Instead, I thought: *I love my body just the way it is. It's gone through so much and it keeps on working.*

Loving my body had to be a demonstration to myself. That's why I joined the fitness challenge in April 2019 and after I won, I never stopped training. The bar kept being raised and I kept going, learning more, finding the right coaches.

When I was younger, diets were punishment and rein-forced a negative self-image. Who hasn't tried to get in shape because of self-disgust? That is not the way. Love yourself and your body right now, just the way you are. Let go of the negative self-talk. Quit saying: "I hate my _____" -(Don't fill in the blank!)

If self-love is hard, try self-acceptance. Be kind to that beautiful soul you are.

When I close my eyes at night, I see a landscape that is part ocean and part sloping hill to the beach. It's twilight, so the sky is a deep purple and blue indigo. There are stars sparkling in the sky. I often see this as a portal to my dreams. It's where for me, transformation takes place. It then takes time for it to manifest out here. But if you hold to what you most desire, infuse it with love and emotion, it will come to pass. Be patient and let it come.

Letter to my donor family:

Dear family of Gina,

If I could tell you what Gina's gift has meant to me, words just are not enough. On the night we got the call that I had an organ donor we know that you were grieving the loss of your loved one, Gina, and that it was unexpected and untimely. It hit me hard that someone had died so that I could live and in the mysterious ways of God, this match I feel was made in heaven. The doctors told me we were so close a blood and antigen match we could have been sisters.

I often try to imagine Gina and send her my love and gratitude. Her mother and I wrote letters for several years but then they stopped and those I sent were returned. My 30th anniversary of the kidney and pancreas (both from Gina) organ transplant came in July, 2021, and I again have a deep desire to express my gratitude to you, her family.

When I went on the organ transplant waiting list, I was 34 and suffering greatly from diabetic complications. My eyes had begun to go blind from proliferative retinopathy, and I had nerve damage throughout my body as well as early-stage heart disease. My blood sugars were up and down like a roller coaster despite my dedication to taking good care of myself. By 34 my kidneys failed and dialysis was one option. Later I was a show-and-tell patient for transplant surgeons at conferences – and I heard the statistics first hand: a diabetic on dialysis had the same prognosis as a person with terminal cancer: five years max. When the hospital said I was a candidate for a kidney transplant and the experimental pancreas transplant I had to think hard about that, because the dual organ transplant would be more difficult to recover from, and I would be under anesthesia for more time. Heart attack and stroke were possible. But I had to take the risk — I could not live the way I had been with the awful disease of diabetes.

So, the call came that night and we sent all our love and prayers to Gina's family – her name was unknown to us at the time – but she or he was a dear soul with a family. I hope you know that I have thought of her and you every day of my life since then. Thirty years.

In those thirty years, I have been so blessed to travel the world, living in Saudi Arabia and Mexico, going to Africa, Sri Lanka, India, Kuwait, Greece, Oman, Morocco, Singapore, Malaysia, Jordan, Italy, Germany, and Spain.

The four years in Saudi Arabia were magical and so was a year in Mexico. I am an artist and I was able to get my Master's Degree in 2018 and I traveled those places to paint and record my experiences.

I have been married to my husband Paul for 32 years and he has stood by me throughout all the health challenges, moves, and adventures we have had together. My transplant came two years into our marriage.

After receiving Gina's pancreas and one kidney, my entire system – blood sugars and kidney function — stabilized within minutes, and over time the retinopathy and nerve damage reversed, even though I have minor floaters in my vision. It took about 14 years for the heart disease to become critical so a triple bypass in 2005 fixed that.

I am now 66 years old and besides God and my parents, Gina gave me life. What a precious gift, what an incredible gift. No one will ever know how transplant patients feel about our donor families and all donor families; you are angels, self-less and giving in a time of deep sorrow and loss – the best of human beings who will reach out to others during incredibly dark and difficult times. You help another while your pain is fresh and raw from deep, unexpected loss.

This letter is so late in coming to you. I hope it reaches you. My life at 66 would not be possible without Gina's gift of her pancreas and one kidney. I live each day hoping that she would know how much I have cherished this gift in how I live my life. In how I love. In how I give and want to serve others in some way.

Inspiration is one way.

In April of 2019, I was living in Mexico with my husband and realized there was so much more I wanted to do in life. Despite relatively good health, there was a little voice inside of me that told me to step it up – I needed to be really fit to continue on this journey of life and do all I wanted and give all I can. So, I started to weight-train. Always athletic as a younger person, I had gotten out of shape and lazy. But I'd think of this gift of life and realize that I had a lot left to do and it's because of Gina.

Within two years, I had reached a status as an athlete working with a trainer to prepare me for a body-building competition. No, not a big bulked-up body, but a strong, lean, vibrant and healthy body – in one that is 64 years young and has organs that are younger than that. I never had more than one simple rejection episode, which was right after the transplant. I have had no trouble at all in 30 years. Is that not an incredible miracle?

The summer of 2021 I placed in two bodybuilding competitions for Masters Bikini age 55 plus and age 60 plus. I share this because it's an inspiration for others to see the incredible transformations and gifts that organ donation affords people who will die without them.

I'm so grateful for my life and that Gina is a part of this miracle means so much to me. I'd love to connect with her remaining family and if we both agree, we can.

On the other hand, if it's not something you want to do, I will completely understand. I would love love love to know more about Gina and hear any memories you have of her.

An organ transplant is so life-affirming. It shows how connected we all are as humans. It's showing the absolute best of human beings, and I hold this sacred thought of you, Gina's family, and of Gina, as a special link to my miracle of life.

With love,
Julia

THE END
(And also, a beginning!)

Postscript:
As of this writing, my donor family has been found and this letter delivered. It was Gina's husband who was found. He was with her in the car when the accident happened that took her life. I don't know the circumstances of the accident, but it's been 30 years since he lost his wife, and I pray he's moved on from painful memories. I have not gotten a response. So, this letter is one that I share with all the donor families who have lost loved ones who went on to give the Gift of Life to another. God Bless you all.

AFTERWORD

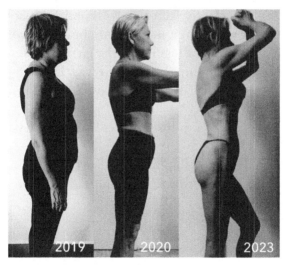

Julia continues to transform

It is never too late and you are never too old to get fit and live a life of amazing energy and joy. There are steps to take to get there and it can seem overwhelming. And it is because there is incredible nuance to the fitness journey. You can take it as far and as long as you like until you get the results you want.

And what you did to get to a fit state, you must continue to do to stay in a fit state.

Here is a breakdown of things that make the fitness journey for the Queenager (50+ in age) very doable and successful.

HOW DO I START? (Most asked question)

MINDSET!
- Commit to a sacred pact with yourself
- Write down your Dream List
- Start with self-love. If that's hard, self-worthiness
- Throw out perfection
- Realize this will take time and patience
- SEE & BE the amazing person you were meant to be, infuse this vision with emotion & belief
- Replace negative self-talk with positive mantras
- Go for the highest in optimum health, however long it takes (weight loss is not the goal, it's a side effect)
- Don't let anything get in your way. Life will test you.
- Let go of what isn't serving you and isn't prioritizing your health
- Make daily mindful choices, not habitual, unconscious ones
- Love your body no matter what state it is in
- Find a fitness tribe to be supported by and to support
- Be consistent
- Quit looking for a quick fix

EXERCISE
- Set up a small home gym with dumbbells
- Add good loop bands and resistance bands
- Work out in workout clothes
- Do 30 minutes a day five times a week to start
- Alternate upper and lower body strength training
- Do LISS cardio fasted - Low Impact Steady State - it burns fat
- Find a trainer, join a gym (gyms offer training)
- Make the time
- Log ALL your workouts, track progress, keep lifting a little heavier each time

- Take progress pics from day one: front, side and back - same pose, bathing suit and lighting
- Track your weight but don't be scale focused – fluctuations are normal
- If you gain 2-5 lbs. in a day know that fat doesn't come on that fast — it's due to something else which is temporary
- Tape measure your waist, hips, and thigh and track changes – you'll see wins here before the scale changes
- Allow your body the time needed to respond to lifestyle changes
- It took me four months to lose the first 10 lbs.

NUTRITION
Prioritize protein for fat loss and muscle building, eat complex carbs, leafy green plants, and healthy fats. The best diet is the one you can sustain long term (with treats here and there!) Ask yourself: could I be eating like this in five years? If no, find another nutrition plan.

COACHING
Julia is certified by the International Sports Sciences Association (ISSA) as a personal trainer. She offers programs for women, age 50 plus, who want to get in the best shape of their life in peri- and post-menopause. Her signature program is the FABULOUS AFTER 50 BLUEPRINT.
For more information go to:
Bodybeautylovelife.com
Or follow her on Instagram @dolphinine and YouTube

FREE E-BOOK
Download Julia's FREE e-book:
FIVE MISTAKES WOMEN MAKE THAT KEEP THEM FROM LOOKING AND FEELING FABULOUS AFTER 50 and How To Fix Them Forever, Step by Step
https://bodybeautylovelife.com/fabulous/download/

ABOUT THE AUTHOR

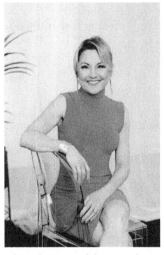

Julia Linn (b. 1957) is a fitness influencer, wellness expert, coach, motivational speaker, and a badass bodybuilder. She has reimagined what it is to be a senior citizen at age 66.

She has lived all over the world as a professor and instead of retiring at 62 she decided to get fit, expressing gratitude for the gift of life an organ transplant gave her. The physical transformation was profound – but more so on the inside where you couldn't see it. It led her to compete onstage in bodybuilding competitions for 60+ and becoming a certified personal trainer and mindset coach. She wants women in their 50s, 60s, and 70s to learn how to think differently about menopause, their bodies, and the toxic culture of weight loss. Because she says, "The world needs your bright light which cannot sparkle and shine unless you feel well."

Photo by @angelahopperphoto

She teaches the principles of transformation and self-reinvention through mindset, training and nutrition coming from a place of self-love and gratitude for your body, not by a disgusted-by-my-body mindset.

The goal is the long game of optimal health, a sustainable lifestyle in which weight loss becomes a happy side effect but is not the goal.

Julia is certified by the INTERNATIONAL SPORTS SCIENCES ASSOCIATION (ISSA) as a Personal Trainer and Coach. Her career includes 40+ years as an educator at the university level. She has given keynote talks and led workshops at spiritual seminars across the globe on personal development since 1994.

She founded **body beauty love life**™ to coach women age 50 and over online from anywhere in the world.

Her message:

The goal is not weight loss, but health.

It's not a desperate hurry to stop hating yourself based on body disgust. It's changing the small stories we tell about ourselves.

It's starting from loving yourself & accepting however long it takes to transform. Because there is no endpoint. Health is your forever goal. If I can do this, you can do this too.

Julia Linn can be found on Instagram @dolphinine, youtube. com/@julialinn and her website www.bodybeautylovelife.com.

Made in the USA
Las Vegas, NV
18 January 2024

84511424R10164